Becoming a Slave

The Theory and Practice of Voluntary Servitude

By Jack Rinella

with Reflections by His Slave Patrick

Published by
Rinella Editorial Services
4205 North Avers Avenue
Chicago, IL 60618 USA

www.RinellaEditorial.com

Cover design by
Michael Tallgrass

Library of Congress Control Number: 2005906150

ISBN 0-940267-20-9

Printed in the United States of America

To my devoted slaves

Patrick & Matthew

And

In memory of our good friend John B. Feuer

And another true slave

rodtney Jordan-ross

Table of Contents

Introduction

It takes as much energy to wish as it does to plan.[*]

I found my first introduction to master/slave (M/s)[†] relationships in the pages of *Mr. Benson*, a novel by John Preston published in 1983. Like *The Story of O* (1954), *Tarnsman of Gor* (1967), and *The Claiming of Sleeping Beauty* (also 1983), fiction has long provided the erotic gist that feeds the imagination of would-be dominants and submissives alike.

But I am not a New York millionaire like Mr. Benson, a prince in an ancient country, a French maiden, or a man transported across the solar system. So, like the rest of us, I have found ways to translate fiction into some kind of satisfactory reality — one not crafted by writers or actors, but by real men and women living in the here and now. I have had to find the master within, while searching for that special person who believes that he or she was not only born to serve, but born to serve me.

This has been a twenty year journey, during which I have met hundreds of people, either in cyberspace or real time: masters and their slaves, serious seekers and flakes, the curious and the experienced. I have attempted to enthrall more than a hundred of them and have been successful, in the short-term, with more than several. My more than nine years with my slave Patrick have proven the viability of my desires, as have the relationships of the masters, mistresses, and their slaves who I have been privileged to know during these years.

Experience shows that M/s relationships are first and foremost human relationships. No amount of domination or submission will change

---

[*] Eleanor Roosevelt, cited in *Whatever It Takes* by Bob Moawad, Compendium Publishing, Lynwood, WA, 2003.

[†] As you read on, you will find that I use M/s and D/s somewhat interchangeably. In fact, both are dominant/submissive relationships. M/s more specifically indicates a master/slave relationship whereas D/s by in itself refers to any dominant/submissive relationship.

the fact that both masters and slaves are human. Intellect, emotion, physical attributes, finances, mores, and morals are part and parcel of our relationships. For that reason, I find that I am too pragmatic for the dogmatists who seek easy, prepackaged solutions for becoming a master or finding a slave. Let me be clear here:

Creating a master/slave relationship is a very personal, completely human activity that will always reflect the unique ideas, preferences, and agreements of the people in the relationship. There is no cookie-cutter recipe for becoming a slave, except that you follow the desires of heart.

An Amazon.com book reviewer once wrote that my work, *The Master's Manual*, might have been written by any marriage counselor in that it was full of common sense suggestions that gave few specific ideas to someone who wanted to be in a dominant/submissive (D/s) relationship. As a friend once said, "Duh." We are humans and relationships between humans will always reflect our humanity.

What is just as true is that even the kinky[‡] aspects of our relationships are seldom consistent and hardly ever universal. I cannot, therefore, give you ready-made presentations as to how you ought to fashion your slave future or, if you are dominant, your future slave. I can paint pictures of broad generalities and give examples of actual practices, but the hard truth is that successful M/s relationships are tailored to the two (or more) people in them. Just as clothes come in many sizes, so too are there wide variations in the M/s continuum. From sadistic tyrant to elegant lady, from chattel farm hand to sissy maid, there is no one style that fits all and no one can easily catalogue all of them either.

I recently read an online post from a writer seeking information about slave protocols — that is, the "rules" by which slaves are to treat their masters and others. She wanted to interview master/slave couples about the correct protocols found in the lifestyle. The interviews that helped shape this book prove that there is no consistent way for M/s relationships to be expressed. Is she looking for protocols between gay Leathermen, between professional Dominatrices and their clients, between elegant mistresses and their attendants, or between sadistic masters and their raunch slaves? Master/slave relationships, after all, come in all sizes, colors, and temperaments.

Even if we examine only one of these modalities, we find wide variations in the specifics. Are slaves supposed to walk in front of their masters, to their right or left, or behind? I can find examples of each practice among those who rightfully identify as master and slave. To

---

‡ For our purposes, kink and kinky refer to any sexual relationship that includes BDSM — that is: bondage, discipline (whipping, spanking, and other impact fetishes), dominance, submission, sadism, and masochism.

label one way better than another is to venture into dangerous territory, to be sure. What I can do is lay down general principles that appear in M/s relationships, while presenting examples that illustrate, rather than directives that limit.

For instance, my friend, Master Vince, has a style of domination quite different from mine. He once met a slave-applicant online and then in person. It seemed to both of them that there was no future between them as master and slave. At the same time, Vince suspected that my style would fit the applicant well and arranged for us to correspond via e-mail. Within the week, the applicant was in my home and eventually was collared and under contract. One style does not fit all.

As a master, I have peculiar ways of doing things and of how I want them done. For better or for worse, you can't create as I have, since you are not me. Imitation may indeed be a compliment, but healthy relationships are built on faithfulness to oneself, not to some idealized fantasy of how one thinks things should be.

My approach in these pages is to clarify and explain, especially by clearly defining and giving actual examples. My aim is to demythologize in order to make attainable a fulfilling master/slave relationship. After all, if you can't live it, it has little purpose beyond feeding one's libido. That's the stuff of porn, not reality. My purpose is to guide you on your very personal path in finding a master, though I trust that masters will also find something of value in this book as well.

A Quick Note about My Writing Style

Contrary to more popular usage, I prefer to use standard American spelling and rules of grammar and punctuation, avoiding (I hope) the more usual misuses of our language. Therefore you will notice that slaves' names begin, as I think they should, with capital letters and that slaves are hes or shes, not its. My reasoning for this is simple: Those who are committed to obey and serve us masters have accepted a high calling, one that I find most honorable and I honor them for doing so. Though many disagree with me (and they have every right to do so), I find the use of the lower case and of impersonal pronouns demeaning. It certainly does nothing to acknowledge the high value I place on what slaves are and what they do. Additionally, nonstandard usage makes a book more difficult to read.

The only places I have been willing to deviate from standard usage are when people asked me to do so when referring to them. Therefore, you will, on occasion, find titles and names in a grammatically incorrect style, but they are after all, their names, not mine.

Several of the readers who proofed the manuscript form of this book pointed out the confusion of similar terms that point to realities that have much in common, yet remain vaguely apart. I admit to using terms interchangeably when, in fact, they refer to distinct, but closely related groups. The interchange of D/s and M/s, of Leather, Lifestyle, and Subculture, and of groups, community, and communities are all just such examples. I do this intentionally, as that allows me to add variety to my writing. Otherwise, if I consistently used the same terms over and over again, I'd be damned for being too repetitious.

In truth, these terms have more things in common than differences, though one can find clear lines of separation, as between gay Leather men and Pansexual munch attendees.§ I will try to define terms that seem to need definition, though I admit that is a value call on my part.

Words as simple as master and slave confuse the discussion. After all, slavery — at least the pre-Civil War kind — is illegal nearly across the planet. What, then, is a slave? The words are found in our literature, our seminars, our classifieds, our films, and our e-mails ad nauseam.

Experience has shown that few are slaves, even fewer masters, if we but look at the words as found in a dictionary.¶ Rather than lump all dominants into a nice neat pile of masters and all submissives as slaves (and many are not), we had best see the terms modified by adjectives, such as wannabe, trainee, applicant, apprenticed, or actual.

The reason I modify the word slave is simple. Used alone, it defines a person who is in a relationship. Just as husband and wife are terms used for those who are actually married, so too does slave reflect a living relationship that is being lived in the current time. Wannabe husbands and wannabe wives are called fiancés and fiancées; they may be engaged, but they are not yet wed. Even on the day of their marriage, we name them bride and groom. Only after the official pronouncement is made are they husband and wife. Likewise, divorced or widowed spouses are no longer called husband or wife.

I know that many of my readers will protest my limited qualification of who is a slave. They really believe they are slaves even though they haven't found a master to serve. Still, I stand my ground on this issue. Be a slave-applicant, or a slave trainee, or say you want to be a slave. The title slave will be much more meaningful and real if you wait and use it when it's truly appropriate.

---

§ A munch is a public meeting of kinky folks, usually held at a restaurant, as a safe way for online people to meet. The munches are places to find play partners, learn about groups, and become part of a real-time and place community. Pansexual means open to all genders and orientations. Gay Leathermen, on the other hand, generally meet in bars, at club functions, or online.

¶ I use the dictionary to provide some understanding to our use and misuse of terms. If, as is often the case, we each use the same word when it means different things to each person in the conversation, we have a serious communication problem.

Let me consider each word individually.

Wannabes

Though the word wannabe has certain unfavorable connotations,[**] we can simply say that a person with no connection to a master, but who is considering slavery as a life option, is a wannabe slave. For them, slavery is an unrealized idea that reflects a potential. We all begin as wannabes, since wanting to be is the beginning of the process. It is first desire that leads us to explore slavery, eventually leading us to become trainees, apprentices, applicants, and, hopefully, slaves.

Trainees

So, I choose to call a person studying or working with a mentor, or potential partner, a slave trainee. Trainees are those learning from a mentor, a person who is simply a casual teacher, or one who is preparing the other to enter into a relationship with them. Apprentices are similar, of course, but I would say that an apprentice is learning from one in order to be in a relationship with someone else. Thus, one master may agree to take on another who wants to be apprenticed as a slave. In this regard, anyone with experience can train or mentor another. In fact, there is great historical precedence for slaves mentoring or training other slaves.

Applicants

When two people agree to the possibility of becoming partners, I consider them to be applicants. Therefore, the master is applying to become the other's master and the slave is applying to become the dominant's property — which will be explained more clearly in later chapters. Until the collar is locked or the contract signed, or however they want to establish the beginning of their relationship, they are applying for a position not yet achieved. Lord knows, there's many a slip between the cup and the lip.

Slaves

Lastly, we need to understand the term "slave." In fact, it is only a shorthand for one who surrenders, obeys, and gives service to one who has the ability and consent to control them. For that reason, it is not altogether correct to use the term slave. As indicated in the subtitle of this book, the actual relationship is better called one of voluntary

---

[**] "Wannabe" has a somewhat negative connotation. I would prefer to use a different term. I can't, for the life of me, come up with a better one. In fact, the word is only a variation of "wants to be," and there is nothing wrong with that.

servitude. Nevertheless, our D/s community continues to call one in just such a relationship "a slave."†† Perhaps, some day, published dictionaries will get on the bandwagon with us and add our definition as well.

The word slave describes an individual who is in that relationship. Getting there is a process of self-knowledge and mutual testing until the partners arrive at an agreed upon dominant/submissive relationship. Just as non-kinky partners court, so too do we — each trying to woo the other. It is a matter of getting to know one another, of testing to see if a relationship could actually work, of understanding each other's aspirations, and the viability of developing a long-term relationship.

The Approach I Take

This book is a blueprint for enthrallment. I will begin with a broad and general definition of the slave, followed by suggestions for finding a master, and concluding with reflections on a slave's life. It is first and foremost factual technique, the alchemy of changing one's current way of life into something still only imagined, one path among many to becoming a slavishly devoted servant. Because our M/s relationships are fully personalized by our own desires and circumstances, you will find that the lessons found herein are full of suggestions and alternatives for designing, creating, and living your personal D/s relationship, rather than an exact plan for accomplishing your M/s goals. In the end, I can only point you in a direction. You and your partner, or partner-to-be, will have to create your relationship for yourselves.

Let me separate fact from fiction. Like most of those experienced in M/s relationships, I find that I spend a lot of time debunking the myths and prejudices that are deeply, and by nature, intertwined within the fantasies of those just entering this lifestyle. Herein are no instructions on reliving the glory that was Rome or Greece, the shame of pre-Civil War slavery, or some fantasy of kidnapping and captivity. Instead, this book is meant to be a guide to voluntary servitude, which is a much more appropriate term for that in which we Leather‡‡ dominants and submissives are so deeply engaged.

This type of relationship holds no escape from life. In fact, like all relationships, it will tend to magnify the areas in your life which need to change. This is no free ride, either for master or slave, as the cost of living is the same: insurance, medical bills, rent, utilities, clothing, education, room and board, vacations, retirement, and all the necessities

†† Throughout this book I will use the term "slave" as a convenient shorthand for the title given a person who is in a relationship of voluntary servitude.

‡‡ "Leather" is used here as a general concept for any and all kinds of kinky relationships, including BDSM, D/s, and alternate lifestyles.

of reality remain. It's not all sex either. It is most likely that more time will be spent outside of the relationship — at work — than in any other place. Then, sleep will consume another third of your week, and most of the rest of the time will be needed for laundry, house cleaning, cooking, shopping, and a host of other assorted chores.

Just deciding to become a slave isn't enough, as you will find the search for your dominant partner will be long and arduous. It will be filled with a great many dead ends, broken promises, and dreamers who will waste your time. Think about it for a minute. One doesn't decide to become a doctor and begin practicing medicine the next day. We don't decide we want a husband or wife and immediately walk down the aisle with the first person we date. Creating a new life path, whatever it might be, takes time, learning, practice, reflection, and (usually) a great deal of preparation. But for those who persevere, a delightful and fulfilling relationship awaits.

The rule here is that the practical and the pragmatic will take precedence over the frivolous and the imaginary. If it doesn't work, we won't use it. If it ain't broke, we won't fix it. We are talking about real lives, lived in a real world. Unlike Mr. Benson, we'll have to go to work (though, to be fair, he did disappear from his penthouse on a daily basis). Unlike Beauty, no prince will awaken us with a kiss and take us to his realm of sexual enthrallment. The relationship described herein is meant to be real, lived daily by real men and women, in real places around the world.

There are two aspects to the journey of becoming a slave: the first is nature; the second is nurture.

By nature, I mean that being submissive has much to do with one's personality and disposition; hence, we talk about being "born to serve." Nature implies certain innate talents, abilities that are part and parcel of who we are.

But nature alone is not enough. Hence, there is a need for nurturing — as in "to educate, to train; to help grow or develop; cultivate."§§ The purpose of this book, then, is to train: "To coach in or accustom to a mode of behavior or performance; to make proficient with specialized instruction and practice." I use "train" purposefully, since real slavery and true service are manifest in behavioral outcomes. Not only are a master and slave who they are, but more importantly, they are known as who they are by how they live and what they do.

For that reason, this book isn't about daddies, tops, bottoms, or submissives, per se, though I surely trust those who identify as such will find much of value in these pages. I admit to being verbally rigorous

§§ All references to definitions are from *American Heritage Dictionary*, Houghton Mifflin, Boston, MA, 1982, unless otherwise noted.

here. I have a rather intense, deeply committed, and serious relationship in mind when I write about mastery and slavery. It's not that those who want to play at it can't, or that the merely curious won't find much of value in my writing. I only state this warning now so that my purpose is clear:

This book is a guide to becoming a slave in devotion and service to a master.

I have also based this book's premise on the assumption that my reader has more than a passing familiarity with our kinky community. The merely curious will find a great deal herein that describes our lifestyle, but I am presuming that my reader is already familiar with the more general customs, mores, and practices found in kinky communities.

In other words, there are basic techniques, modes of communication, and a unique vocabulary that probably ought to be learned before one decides to enter into a long-term master/slave relationship.

Your understanding of masters and slaves needs be rooted in a familiarity with the general culture of Leather, as learned by your full participation within that community. If you haven't yet met "us" in the real world, I suggest you read a primer¶¶ or two, and find a Leather bar or club, a munch or monthly play party; become an active participant in our lifestyle before you seek a master. Mastery and slavery are no places for a lone ranger, if only because you're going to have to meet a lot of people before you meet the one meant for you.

Ideally, one trains through a wide variety of activities. I will be the first to admit that just reading this book isn't going to make you a slave. One needs the experience of sharing with those who have relevant experience, perhaps even being mentored by them, of practicing specific activities and behaviors associated with service. Only when they occur naturally in one's daily life is it possible to decide how to express and arrange your life and its relationships in real ways that allow you to be a slave. Nuances of method and execution, of speech, and of thought must be understood. The road to attaining full maturity in one's chosen lifestyle includes undergoing psychological and emotional changes.

Both mastery and service will be naturally structured by the two (or more) people in the relationship. Your very personal histories, personalities, localities, orientations — among a host of other

¶¶ I suggest my *Partners in Power*, Greenery Press, Oakland, CA, 2003. Appendix D lists others.

characteristics — determine who you are and what you want to be. You can't submerge who you are or from whence you came in the living of a relationship. For that reason, there is neither one way to be a master, nor one way to be a slave. When lived to its fullest, it will be your (and this word is plural) creation. What I can give you in these pages are guidelines, suggestions, and real life examples upon which you can model your own beliefs, desires, and behaviors.

The greater part of this book is derived from my 20-plus years of mastery, including five years as a slave. The book also incorporates information from interviews with men and women who have experience in a master/slave relationship. I have tried to be as comprehensive as possible, including both men and women of all orientations and lifestyles. Each has lived in a committed master/slave relationship for at least one year. That, and the willingness to be interviewed, were the only criteria for inclusion.

I have also interviewed several others who attempted to create this kind of relationship without success, thereby giving some examples and fostering an understanding of what might be avoided.

About Patrick's Reflections

At the end of each chapter you'll find reflections from Patrick, my 24/7 slave of nine years. They are his heartfelt and experienced-based thoughts on life in voluntary servitude. Like me, you will find him a happy, intelligent, and contented individual. His strength has strengthened me. Here, his thoughts strengthen my words.

For those who are curious, Patrick is nine years younger than I, has a Master's degree in Community Development, and presently works full-time outside our home as Business Development Manager for a video and book distribution company. We own our home jointly and in it he cares for me daily as cook, shopper, janitor, butler, laundry guy, and fabulous sex partner. He is also active in one of our local Leather clubs and spends much of his free time reading Star Trek novels.

In discussing the writing of his reflections, we had to arrive at what he should call me in print. We settled on "Sir," since that is his usual form of address to and about me. Though I am somewhat wary of titles, such as "My Sir," I accept the title Sir from him as a shorthand that acknowledges my mastery of him and his surrender to me. I trust you will see that word in the same light and, therefore, appropriate for his use. You, on the other hand, are certainly free to call me "Jack."

Acknowledgements

Few books are solo endeavors. Therefore, I wish to acknowledge the hundreds of men and women who have taught me the way of mastery and service, especially Master Lynn and slave Patrick. The masters and slaves who graciously allowed me to interview them for source information and the examples you find in this book also deserve my thanks: Master Jim & slave Marsha (International Master & slave 2001, a gay and lesbian couple), Steve Sampson & slave Kirk (International Master & slave 2000), Master Vince DiFruscio (a longtime friend in Chicago), Master Scott & Slavette (International Master & slave 2002 and husband and wife), Goddess Lakshimi (Professional Dominatrix with a 24/7 slave and Ms. World Leather 2004), and Master Lawrence & slave Ernest (a gay couple).

I would also like to acknowledge and thank those who were kind enough to read this manuscript in its early form and offer suggestions and corrections: TammyJo Eckhart, Joanne Gaddy, Phil Ross, and slaves Patrick, Marsha, and Slavette.

As I end this introduction, I strongly urge you to do the "After Reading Activities." This book is meant to help you on your journey; if you are only talking and not walking, you'll never arrive there. The activities' intent is to help you reflect on the readings to provide a better understanding of what you want.

When you do the exercises, you will create an actual journal with three purposes: First, it will have samples of letters, questions, and answers that you will want to have handy for your prospective master. Doing so will be a good way to show your seriousness, while providing a springboard to discussion. Secondly, you will have done your homework, by creating a personal ad and a petition. Thirdly, you will have a personalized guide with questions and answers for your interviews.

Finding a master is a journey. Good luck and as we sang in my childhood, "Happy trails to you."

Patrick Reflects: First Thoughts

Being a slave has a lot to do with feeling. It *feels* good to serve. There is general contentment in being where you belong and a satisfaction at being bold enough to allow yourself to achieve it. Physical contact with the one you serve is joyous and the attention you are shown causes you to beam with further joy. An intimate little world develops; you can explore each other in ways you never imagined and in ways others can't conceive.

Those feelings are not fleeting, as they are when you are caught up in the fantasy of slavery, when certainty lasts only until orgasm. The feelings I refer to remain and build upon each other, growing stronger and more secure with the passage of time. When a master/slave relationship is successful, these feelings are ongoing; a bond is created with your Master that transcends the chain that might be around your

10

neck or the contract that you might have signed.

That's what it feels like to be a slave, and you can't feel that way wishing for it or fantasizing about it. And I'm sorry, folks, you can't experience it online. You have to *become* a slave to experience such feelings and that's what this book is about: a guide to finding your way to fulfillment through voluntary servitude.

The first thing you will have to do is overcome your fear. Even if you've wanted it all of your life, when the moment of truth is at hand, part of you resists. Fear grabs hold of your logic and manufactures reasons and excuses for why you can't follow your desires just quite yet. Shame can enter into it, as well. We're talking about erotic submission and both of those words are counter to what we are taught is appropriate. This resistance to our desires occurs time and time again, sometimes for years. And when you do begin to make positive steps to pursue your desire, the resistance can even get stronger. This exchange between desire and fear continues until the desire and longing to be who you really are can no longer be held back, and you conquer your fear and take those first real steps.

This first real step I refer to is different for everyone, but you know it has happened by the way your determination moves you in a purposeful way. It may not be the step that transforms your life instantly, but a first step can always be followed by more steps.

That first real step *feels* wonderful. There is a certainty in knowing you are headed to where you belong. Others won't understand it, but they can't be expected to; they aren't on such a path. It feels right even in the midst of not knowing precisely what's ahead.

But the journey to becoming a slave, no matter how "right" and "natural" it feels, isn't easy or instantaneous. Like the young wolf that Jack London wrote of in *White Fang*, there will be resistance even in the midst of growing certainty that this is what is right for you.

> *It came hard, going as it did, counter to much that was strong and dominant in his own nature; and, while he disliked it in the learning of it, unknown to himself he was learning to like it. It was a placing of his destiny in another's hands, a shifting of the responsibilities of existence. This in itself was compensation, for it is always easier to lean upon another than to stand alone....But it did not all happen in a day, this giving over of himself, body and soul, to the man-animals.****

A true slave never loses his strength or dominance. Erotic slavery

*** London, Jack, *The Call of the Wild, White Fang, & To Build a Fire*, Random House, New York, 1998, p. 148

isn't about being beaten into submission. Quite the contrary, you retain those good parts of yourself and turn them to helping you serve your Master, and that's when the journey becomes exciting and fulfilling. Your strength and dominance become tools that help you serve better.

Commitment to this path is a weighty thing, however. When fear takes hold and causes panic at the thought of continuing, the easy way out is to run and deny yourself. If slavery is indeed your destiny, such fears will subside. Eventually, your thoughts will return to what you really want and you will continue your journey.

There is another feeling that is important to talk about at this point in our discussion: loneliness. In society, you can be in the midst of a crowd and still be overwhelmed by loneliness. You can be surrounded by a loving family and friends and still feel alone because you don't believe they really understand who you are. Loneliness can come about as a result of feeling overwhelmed by responsibilities, or dissatisfaction with life, or by forcing yourself to live up to someone else's expectations. I think many people want to become a slave simply because they want someone to love them, to cherish them for who they are.

Whatever the form of loneliness, becoming a slave is not the ultimate solution. It is an illusion to think it entails giving up all control and responsibility, and hiding from the outside world, being taken down to your raw self, and remade into whatever will make you be valued; this isn't slavery. You first need to face whatever it is that is causing your loneliness and conquer it — coming out of the experience a more confident person and better able to discern if slavery is to be a part of your future.

Books about slavery are often written by masters. While they certainly have a clear understanding about what slavery involves, their understanding is based on an opposing perspective: dominance (i.e., having a slave and being served). Slaves qualified to write on the subject are busy serving their masters and would rather do so than spend time writing about HOW they serve. So, the task is usually left to the masters and so many important nuances are left out. Hopefully, that will change as other experienced slaves and their masters realize the importance of contributing to our unique community the experiences they gathered and the lessons they've learned.

When my Master, Jack Rinella (who did live five years as a slave to Master Lynn), decided to write a book on becoming a slave, he encouraged me to consider making some contributions in the form of reflections for each chapter. Sometimes, these are based on the general topic of the chapter, sometimes on a specific idea in a chapter, and sometimes my comments were only prompted by memories of how that topic has played out in my own relationship. But all of them are insights I offer out of my own experience and observations. I hope you will respect them as such, and use them on your journey, if they are helpful.

I should also mention here that I use proper capitalization for my name and the pronoun "I," at my master's request. He says the nuns slapped his hands hard enough to teach him proper usage and his preference is that I do the same. He slaps my butt and face for other reasons.

Becoming a Slave: The Theory and Practice of Voluntary Servitude will be a good companion to your journey. Use it to help you understand the many feelings this journey will bring.

After Reading Activities

Get yourself a loose-leaf notebook, or start a word processing document, in which you will keep a journal. Use the journal to write about your first contact with the idea of slavery. Was it in a book? A movie? From a friend? How did you feel about it then? How do you feel about it now? Why do you find it attractive? Why are you reading this book? Why do you want to be a slave? These questions can lead to greater understanding of yourself and give you some answers for those master applicants wise enough to ask them of you.

What myths and assumptions about slavery do you think you have that might not be based on reality? Can you describe your greatest obstacle to finding a dominant partner? What assets do you think you bring to such a relationship?

If you meet regularly with like-minded friends, you might want to bring this book to a meeting and share a paragraph or two from this chapter. How do others react to the questions above?

1

A Complementary Relationship

In trying to speak in generalities, I know I am going to run headlong into the exceptions, with the inevitable result of someone pointing out an example that doesn't fit. As I've noted before, human beings are far too variable to be classified into watertight compartments.*

When it comes to M/s relationships, appearances can be most deceiving, probably because most people view this relationship through eyes (and with a mind) tainted by the myths of fiction. To the unknowing, our lifestyle appears unequal, unfair, and unlivable. In fact, successful M/s relationships are based upon mutual support and the benefits that each partner receives from being in the relationship. Without mutual gratification, this relationship, as any other, will quickly sour and end — at least as a satisfying relationship — if not in reality.

We can also look at this by thinking of our "bottom line."† What must you have in a relationship in order to be fulfilled? This question also addresses limits and will be discussed in greater depth as the book develops.

Mutuality isn't the same as equality; so, the partners' support of one another may be expressed differently, but mutually. The differences between the partners' roles are complementary, so that each gives to the other in such a way that each is empowered by, and satisfied in, those roles. It is important to point out that the word "mutual" means,

---

* Townsend, Larry, *The Leatherman's Handbook,* The Traveller's Companion, Inc., New York, 1972.

† Thanks to Slavette for this addition.

15

"Having the same relationship each to the other; Directed and received in equal amount." Therefore, in the context of this discussion, there can be no such thing as a master/slave relationship in which one partner gives or takes "more" than the other. One can only give as much as the other is willing to receive. One cannot be more of a master, for instance, unless the partner is willing to become more of a slave.

Your search for a partner is actually the search for your complement, that special person whose temperament and vision for his or her future fits with yours. The characteristic of "fitness" is what allows the relationship to work. It is also the reason that finding one's partner is so difficult. You both must fit, and fitting involves a wide spectrum of characteristics, be they physical, intellectual, social, economic or fantastic — meaning that your fantasies are complementary as well.

I hope it's obvious that fantasy plays an important part in one's desire to become a slave. For that reason, I called one of the characteristics listed above "fantastic." Fantasy, by itself, is very often ultimately unattainable. Nevertheless, when viewed as part of our imagination, it feeds our creativity, providing gist for a vision toward which we can work; by doing so, we eventually arrive at a transformation of some part of that fantasy into reality.

In fact, the purpose of this book is to facilitate transformation — that is, "an act or instant of transforming." To transform is "to change markedly the form or appearance of; to change the nature, function, or condition of." In short, this is a book about change.

Change is probably the most necessary condition one must embrace in order to create a master/slave relationship. Change, too, is always with us — the natural state of human existence. Every minute of our lives we age, and therefore, we change. More specifically, we must start with the question of, "How do I have to change to be what I want to become?" How will you be different when you are a slave? What actions and decisions will, in fact, transform you from who you are now to what you seek to become?

Over the more than twenty years that I have been seeking slaves, I have seen innumerable instances where resistance to change has been the strongest obstacle to realizing the applicant's goal. This resistance is most often manifest not in speech, but in action, or perhaps it might be better said that it is manifest in inaction.

How many readers, I wonder, skipped over the "After Reading Activities" at the end of the introduction? Reading about becoming a slave will not train you to be a slave. You must embrace the transformational process by action. Let me state again that real-time slavery and true service are manifest in behavioral outcomes. If you are willing to be trained as a slave, you must be willing to change your actions so that

16

they reflect slavery. You must divest yourself of those things which keep you from your stated goal and acquire those skills and artifacts that will allow you to act as a slave.

In most cases, this is not as serious a step as your fear and doubt would have you believe. We are talking about small, reasonable steps at every step of the journey. Much of this book, in fact, is about those steps. The task is to make yourself ready, prepared for the future about which you now dream.

An important step in creating a successful M/s relationship is to find that part of your fantasy which can be created and to acknowledge that which will never become real, shedding it in some measure from your vision, if not your dream life. For that reason, one's search — though sired and fed by fantasy — must be rooted in the possible. What's possible, of course, is incredibly varied. It is possible to find a partner with the wherewithal to fulfill a fantasy for long-term confinement, for instance. Whether or not that is *probable* is another story, but probability must also be taken into account. So, possibility must be weighed with probability and the true seeker for a master will do all he or she can to improve the probability of success.

Refine your fantasy into a practical vision about yourself, your partner-to-be, and your future life together. By looking at your M/s relationship in terms of reciprocal characteristics, you can evaluate your fitness for each characteristic, and thereby gain an understanding of your future partner's characteristics as well.

There are a large number of attributes we can consider and I am certain that there's no way I can list and explain all of them. In fact, such a list could be self-defeating, as none of us has a crystal ball foretelling what the future will hold when it comes to partnerships. The first caveat, then, is to keep your vision flexible and your options open. History is a strong indicator that the person who you least expect, when you least expect it, will present him or herself as an almost perfect fit. No one is perfect, but "almost" is certainly better than no one.

In all of this, I have to emphasize the necessity of what I call "clicking," an especially important attribute. It is that elusive quality of knowing that the other is just right. The knowing is part intellectual, part emotional, part physical, and part generally indescribable. Without reason, though there may be lots of reasons, the other is the one with whom you click — and you know that all fantasy, reason, and pragmatism will give way for you to accommodate him or her into your life.

What each of my partners have shared is that, for various reasons, they all had qualities that made them just right, even if they didn't have the qualities that I was seeking. For that matter, when I met most of them,

I wasn't even seeking a relationship. That is certainly the case with Master Lynn, who I met for a simple scene and ended serving for five years. When we met, I instinctively knew he would make a wonderful partner — and he did. It was a matter of the right chemistry, at the right time.

Authority and Obedience

The primary characteristics in the M/s relationship are the complementary attributes of authority and obedience. Unlike more common relationships, where these two factors are relegated under other characteristics such as love, finances, or friendship, the master and slave are wont to structure their lives within these two attributes: the master recognizing, acknowledging, and exercising authority over his slave, who grants him or her that position; likewise, the slave pledges, desires, and practices obedience as that which is due to his or her master.

Herein the complementary nature of the relationship is most clearly seen. The master can have no more authority than the slave is willing to grant by the act of his act of submission and the manifestation of his or her obedience. Without obedience, authority is meaningless. Without authority there is no one to obey.

In the final analysis, it is the degree to which authority is exercised and obedience given that determines the quality and the depth of the M/s relationship. It's not that other relationships don't have aspects of authority and obedience, as they most certainly do. What is unique about this relationship is the primacy of these two attributes. It's here, of course, that the greatest amount of misinformation abounds. Few, for instance, understand the degree to which authority may be demanded, expected, and expressed, especially when obedience is sought outside of the context of sexual gratification.

Many, on the other hand, think that obedience is only meant as a role-playing game, that authority comes without responsibility, or that the exercise of authority is without restraint. As we'll see in later chapters, all characteristics of human relationships have limits. Such is the case here as well.

There are many other complementary characteristics: domination and service, sadism and masochism, receiving and giving pleasure, control and surrender, and adoration and devotion to name but a few. The importance and energy each couple places on each of these characteristics all play a part in creating and determining the kind of relationship you have.

As we shall see, control and surrender are expressions of authority and obedience. Sadomasochism may or may not be part of the M/s relationship. Both master and slave will have to give and receive, though in different ways.

When considering M/s relationships, start with my tried and true generalization: **Every relationship is defined by the two (or more) people in the relationship.** I know that we would all like to have ready-made, one size fits all, rules for being master and slave, but life just isn't that way. It is the right of every kinky person to decide how to live his life. Everyone, with his partner, creates a unique relationship.

The way some people pontificate, you'd think that wasn't the case. Dogmatism has no place in our lifestyle. While we certainly all should heed the words safe, sane, and consensual, even they give us a wide berth for playing and determining what those words mean for us as individuals.

I purposefully used the word "people" because both tops and bottoms can be dogmatic. Many call themselves master when they control no one, sometimes not even themselves. Even in a scene, they have no authority to move their bottoms to action for any length of time. Fetish play, being a mutually enjoyable activity — we hope! — hardly involves control. In fact, it is often the bottom, with his infamous safe word, who is in control. The top, in reality, "serves" the bottom's needs by participating in the fetish.

Like the word slave, the word master refers not to a sexual position or inclination, but to one who is in a relationship with a slave. Anyone can be a top. It takes two to make a master.

Dominance and Submission

My dictionary gives me a rather clear place to start when it comes to the word dominance: "The condition or fact of being dominant." Well, OK, maybe it's not that clear; so, let me look down the page for the word dominant: "Exercising the most influence or control; governing; most prominent in position or prevalence."

This is the essence of the M in M/s. Notice that there is no mention of power or pain. Those aspects will have to be negotiated when you mutually determine how broad the influence is and how much control is exercised. It is really about granting your master or mistress first place, though not necessarily having that relationship with the rest of the folks in the dungeon.

Looking elsewhere in the dictionary, we see that submission is, "The act of submitting to the power of another; the state of having submitted." Refining the definition further by looking at the word submit, we find that it means, "To yield or surrender (oneself) to the will or authority of another." Those words are more to my liking and closer to the point of what we expect in M/s.

I think it's noteworthy to see that while M/s does involve the exchange of power, the exchange is more precisely begun by the submissive, not the dominant. Note that in the definition of the word dominance, the word "most" is a qualifier. The submissive exercises influence and control in the relationship as well. The operative word in the definition of the word submit is surrender. In my experience, it is the act of surrender and the degree to which it takes place that creates the D/s relationship. For me, that means that the dominant is not the aggressor so much as he or she is the recipient. Dom(mes) don't take power. They receive it. This understanding puts the relationship on a very sound basis, one that is entirely consensual.

This line of thinking brings me to another word I used a great deal in *Partners in Power: continuum* — that is, "A continuous extent, succession, or whole no part of which can be distinguished from neighboring parts except by arbitrary division." Yes, we would like to have clear-cut distinctions between masters, doms, tops, and daddies (of any and all genders and orientations), but such is not to be. The continuum stretches from the most demanding dictator, to the most permissive top. Your D/s relationship can be strict or easygoing, intense or carefree, temporary or long-term, all the time (often called 24/7), or only when scheduled. You see, I'm going to retreat to my previous statement: It is up to the two (or more) of you to determine what works for you.

For example, there is a well-known master/slave couple who cause many of us to shake our heads. The slave is loud, aggressive, and to the casual observer, appears to be the one in control. Who are we to judge? If they enjoy their relationship (and they certainly do), that is what matters.

To clarify the nature of D/s, it's helpful to remember that top and bottom are positions; they do NOT necessarily determine dominance or submission. We can too easily fall into a category trap: labeling what we do with simplistic words that indicate an act, without analyzing the act's intent. Topping, after all, can be a very submissive act and bottoms can be very much in control. That's one of the reasons that M/s can be so confusing. What you see may not be what is happening.

If we refine our dictionary search further, we can turn to the pages where we find master: "A person having control over the action of another or others," and slave: "One bound in servitude to a person or household as an instrument of labor." Going a bit further in today's vocabulary lesson, we find that servitude is "Submission to a master." As a more intense form of D/s, the master/slave relationship, then, is defined by greater control. Note that it is not simply control, but "control over the action of another or others." The M/s relationship can be best evaluated by the extent to which control is expressed in action. Giving a few orders — which may or may not be actually done — over the Internet is certainly a different degree of control than one has over a slave who lives in one's home and performs his or her required actions throughout the day, week, month, and year.

I admit to being a writer, but for me, my D/s has got to involve more than words. Actions speak louder than words in every case and bring greater satisfaction.

In any case, "voluntary servitude" rather than slavery is a more appropriate name to describe our master/slave relationship, since it is both consensual and service-oriented. Words, though, change only slowly and I'm not about to introduce my slave as my volunteer servant. It just doesn't have the same erotic ring to it.

What, then, are the characteristics of a healthy M/s relationship? Which attributes do the master and slave share and which are more appropriately the slave's? Responsibility is certainly a shared attribute, as are trustworthiness, security, satisfaction, and empowerment. Let me take one of these at a time.

Responsibility

I once took a two week trip to my ancestral homes in Sicily; so, my slave, Patrick, was going to be on his own. Knowing that, a friend casually asked if I had appointed a guardian master over him for the duration. Later I joked to Patrick about my absence and told him about the question. He then noted that he had made an adult decision to be my slave and was adult enough to take care of himself when I was gone. "Well said," I thought, when he gave me that response.

Because so much information about the master/slave lifestyle deals with kink and sex and has fiction as its source, there is this myth that we live irresponsible lives. In fact, for folks really involved in our lifestyle (as contrasted to those who only dream), nothing could be further from the truth.

Responsibility is the ability to respond accountably. As adults, we know how to respond appropriately to various situations, keeping our priorities aligned correctly, and our reactions correct (we hope). In that light, there isn't, nor can there be, any abnegation of duty or safety. Sure, we're in this for fun, but we recognize that there is a time and place for everything and we keep everything in its place.

David Stein, one of the authors of the Gay Male SM Activists'[‡] preamble that gave rise to Safe, Sane and Consensual (SSC), notes that the expression was "intended to draw lines between SM behavior we wanted to encourage and other behavior we wanted to distance ourselves

---

‡   A New York based educational group.

from."§ To distinguish our behavior from that which is irresponsible and abusive is a burden that lies upon us all; to foster positive, healthy, and enjoyable sexual activity and to discourage the opposite is up to us. (You'll find more on abuse in chapter nine.)

In this regard, there are many distinctions that may and should be made. Slaves, for instance, are not children when it comes to their ability to decide correctly. As regards the law, one can never renounce their freedom to choose, or his obligation to decide rightly. "Because my master told me to" is never an excuse for misbehavior, carelessness, injury, or the like.

Though fiction feeds the libido, and in some ways instructs imagination, we are still subject to life on this planet, including its legal, moral, social, and physical rules. I am far from being a conformist, but that gives me no right to be dangerous, illegal, or immoral. The truest forms of our lifestyles are honest and trustworthy, neither deceitful nor dangerous.

Though we take risks and play on the edge, we do so with information and appropriate safeguards. We are risk aware and take steps to minimize injury, disease, and contention. We ensure that we are consensual and in control of ourselves and our play, even when we knowingly give that control to another.

Looking at a slave's life, for instance, will most often show a hard-working, conscientious, and caring person, living a life that — in many respects — is much like anyone else's. The myth of captivity in the basement or of continuous bondage is just that, with little substance or basis in reality. Slaves generally work outside the home and have substantial responsibilities domestically as well. Patrick, for instance, as per our agreement, maintains our home, decides our weekly menu, and makes many daily choices that affect how we both live. He works full-time and is also a partner in an online commercial endeavor.

Masters have the responsibilities of chores, employment, and life in general. Just because our stories often take place in the dungeon doesn't mean that the rest of the week doesn't look like anyone else's week. There are appointments to be kept, bills to be paid, and the usual array of necessary chores that are part of most everyone's life. The vast majority of us have to work for a living and have the same problems, concerns, and challenges as any other human on this planet.

I once met an attractive young man at the Eagle, a Leathermen's bar in Chicago. During our conversation, he told me he was new to Leather and, in fact, this was the first time he had ventured out in his new kinky attire. Like each and every one of us when we were newbies, he was still feeling his way around our subculture, exploring and experimenting,

§ Stein, David, "Safe Sane Consensual: The Evolution of a Shibboleth," which can be found on the Internet at "http://www.lthredge.com/ds/history.htm."

trying to find out what we were really all about.

In that conversation, he indicated that he didn't want his involvement in Leather to interfere with the rest of his life, especially his employment. There was this unstated reluctance to throw away everything he was and did in order to be kinky — as if being kinky meant that he would wear chaps and a harness to work. In due time, of course, he will learn that each and every one of us maintains appropriate priorities and decorum, knowing when, where, and how to act according to truthful, honest, and mutually acceptable norms.

The fact of the matter is that we are human in every situation and living an alternate lifestyle does not diminish our humanity. We are doctors, lawyers, teachers, parents and spouses. We are students, unemployed, laborers, clerks and salespeople. We are young and old, ethnically, religiously, culturally, and racially diverse. When you leave out the kinky aspects of our lives, we fall along the bell curve of humanity in the same way as any group of humans. We spend the largest part of the 168 hour week in the same way as any other people do: We sleep, eat, wash, work, and attend to a myriad of domestic, social, and employment obligations.

The daily drudgery of life has no place in hot fiction and steamy porn. Hence, much of our master/slave literature misrepresents our reality. That's not to knock it. Literature is meant to distract, amuse, delight, and give pleasure. In the same way, we look for dungeons, play spaces, and bedrooms to be places for relaxation, pleasure, and renewal. Our goal is, after all, to have fun. We don't want to have the burdens of laundry, dusting, and dishes interfere with a good scene and passionate sex. Happily they need not.

Every once in a while, though, it's good to remind ourselves that we live on a real planet, in a real world, assuring all who seek us out that we are safe, sane, and consensual; we are part and parcel of humanity's totality.

It's helpful, too, to remind ourselves of our humanity, lest we blame our faults and foibles on the fact of our kinkiness. The pest at our munch is probably a pest at home and at work as well. Those among us who are socially awkward — to put it nicely — in the dungeon are most likely to be the same everywhere else. Conceivably, they may be more comfortable there than we are having them there. Sure, our sexual expressions vary from the norm, whatever that means, but for the most part, we are no different than our neighbors, coworkers, and the families that raised us.

Life as an adult brings responsibilities. Being in a D/s relationship will not remove them, despite what one may wish for in fantasy life.

Trustworthiness

As important as trust is in all relationships between humankind, it takes on a greater importance in our kinky relationships. After all who's going to let themselves be tied up by someone they don't trust?

Trust is "confidence in the ability, reliability, and veracity of a person." In that regard, it is easy to see that there are various levels of trust, just as there are degrees of confidence, such as: "I think," "Maybe," "Possibly," "I know," "I'm sure," and "I'm certain." The greater the degree of confidence — that is, the more you trust me — the more you will allow me to do something to you, or the more you will believe what I say. Complementing trust is surrender. The more you feel you can trust me, the more deeply you will surrender to me and to the scene or relationship in general.

Trust says as much about ourselves as it does about the person we are trusting. A novice to the scene, whom I'll call Chuck, and I once spent three hours talking about his confusion. Seems he couldn't make up his mind about SM. It was a long-time fantasy that remained unfulfilled. He just couldn't decide what to do. Unfortunately, this was not a minor problem. In fact, he couldn't make up his mind in many areas of his life. Should he move to a better neighborhood? Go back to school? Find a better job? And if he finds an answer, how will he know it's the right answer?

So, I began talking about trusting yourself. "Isn't it a matter of trusting others, not yourself?" he asked. "Not entirely," I replied. Trusting someone else first depends upon trusting your own perceptions and conclusions. Confusion sets in not only because we don't trust others, but because we don't trust our own ability to decide who is trustworthy. To find someone to trust, we've first got to have faith in our being able to do so. The part of trust that matters is in oneself, since correctly knowing when and who to trust is important.

Notice that there is nothing vague about trust. With the use of that trait, we are noting our partner's ability, reliability, and veracity. The first — ability — speaks to one's technical proficiency; the second, to their commitment; the third, to their truthfulness. All of these qualities, of course, are related. Some folks, for instance, who are relatively unskilled, will exaggerate their abilities. Exaggeration implies a lack of truthfulness. We can, for instance, make some kind of a promise, break that promise and endanger whether someone trusts us.

It's not just bottoms who have to trust, or only tops who have to be trustworthy. This quality applies to both equally. Bottoms, after all, can rip off a top. I once had a slave-applicant talk me into buying him an expensive airplane ticket to Chicago. In the final analysis, he really wanted a ticket to travel to a Chicago-based Leather convention, not to my dungeon. In less expensive scenarios, tops have to trust that their bottoms will give good feedback about a scene, both during and after it. I have to trust that my slave-applicant is really serious in his negotiations with me. He, too, has to know that I am telling the truth.

Becoming trustworthy, like most of life, is a process. Trusting is the same. In both cases, trust must be earned. I know some masters demand it before it's deserved, but it's my humble (OK, not so humble) opinion that these folks are the last ones we should trust. They are using bravado when trustworthiness is necessary. It is trust that proves itself that increases trust and builds confidence in the other.

There is a risk in all of this. I can only note that if one doesn't take calculated risks, then there can never be any progress. It is as simple as nothing ventured, nothing gained. On the other hand, by moving slowly, risk can be limited and the potential for failure significantly reduced. Please note, though, that moving slowly is very different from not moving. Taking a calculated risk is different from taking no risk at all.

How do we decide that we can trust someone? Experience is certainly the best teacher. By living, risking, trying, trusting, and failing, we learn to trust — both ourselves and our applicants. Successful trust, of course, builds more trust. On the other hand, it is often the case that even the smallest experiences with untrustworthiness can imperil the trust that took weeks, months, or years to build.

Familiarity with a person's trustworthiness builds more trust. It is as simple as that. For that reason, I give small, noncommittal tasks to applicants, testing them to see if they can do what I ask. If they agree and don't fulfill, that's a sure sign of their untrustworthiness. It may not end the conversation, but I will certainly challenge their ability to follow directions and gain my trust.

So, I ask a slave-applicant to send me a picture. When I get the picture, I know that there is the beginning of a relationship. Later, I may ask him to find out the fare and schedule for an airplane ticket to visit me. When he responds with a prompt answer, my trust in him increases.

Experience, happily, isn't the only way that trust can be earned. Many of us are trusted simply based on our reputations — an excellent reason to take care that our reputations never become tarnished. Even association can make or break trust. Patrick, for instance, almost ignored my ad searching for a slave, since he held the magazine in which he read it in such low esteem. Fortunately my other writings spoke more loudly in my favor.

References, too, can help you gain someone's trust and demonstrate his trustworthiness. It is a shame that we don't use references, and check them, as much as we once did. To many people, getting references seems nearly impossible, but that is most likely because they have an exaggerated idea of what it means or haven't made the effort to have experiences with those who can later serve as references. A reference is simply one who can vouch for stated facts about you, perhaps someone who has seen you flog another or who has flogged you. We are only looking for one or two individuals who can affirm that you are who you say you are and that you are a safe individual. It need not even be someone in the scene, though a fellow player is probably to be preferred. Anyone who knows you and will comment on your character will do. That is, at least, a start and if they know your character from experience in the scene, that's all the better.

Observation is another way to determine someone's trustworthiness. By observation, we can note their abilities. We can see whether or not they keep their promises. Are they, for instance, prompt in doing what they say they will do? Can you rely on them in the small things, as well as the large? Have you noted their truthfulness, their openness, and their manners? How free are they with information about themselves, their experiences, and their past relationships? People who have something to hide are usually not to be trusted, even if they reveal their secrets to you. After all, if they are cheating on their wives, they'll probably not hesitate to cheat on you. If they can rationalize away a white lie, they'll find reasons to excuse their black ones too. Even those who may have integrity in one part of life can be dishonest in other areas, such as the accountant who keeps books honestly, but cheats on his wife.

I would add that the use of a "screen name" is appropriate, as it provides a method of protecting one's privacy. Once a real dialogue is begun, though, it is probably best if real names be revealed, with the clear understanding that they not be misused.

That's not to say that a trustworthy person tells all. Privacy and discretion are valuable. There is a difference between privacy and secretiveness. Trusting, after all, implies mutual trust. The guideline here is that each partner should look for and give the amount of trust that is appropriate to the relationship, and its longevity and seriousness. A one-scene partner needs much less information than one I am asking to live with me. As I wrote earlier, there are levels of trust and we need only look for that level which is appropriate to the stage or intensity in which our relationship finds itself.

Sometimes, of course, we have to extend a little trust, hoping that we will not be taken advantage of from having done so. We also have to take ability into account; a person may be trustworthy, yet overestimate his abilities to perform that which we trust him to do. Others ought not push trust in us past our abilities either.

Trust grows and it is the task of both participants to nourish it. It continues to grow, even after a relationship matures. Likewise, trust demands lifelong care, lest the time come when our trust is diminished by the small darts of daily living.

Security

Like trust, the ability to inspire security is a necessary quality in M/s relationships. It is only by feeling secure that we can reach the levels of intimacy that are so necessary to a happy life. Rate, therefore, how secure your applicant (whether they be seeking slavery or mastery) makes you feel and make real efforts to increase their sense of security with you.

Though this sense of security is probably more obviously a bottom's requirement, it is not one-sided. Both partners need to make the other feel secure in what is happening, be it in a scene or in a relationship. For that reason, threats — even when made in jest — are dangerous because they can reduce one's feeling of security. Look for ways to make your applicant or your partner feel more secure, not less. It is only then that you will help him or her relax and enjoy what you are sharing.

Security, of course, is another word for safety. Does your applicant make you feel safe by his or her actions, or do they give you a sense of apprehension or misgiving? If your correspondence with a person doesn't make you feel safe, then you need to seriously consider ending the dialogue. Likewise, you need to be sure that your actions make your applicant feel safe and secure as well.

Again, this advice is sometimes not practiced. There is this myth that masters ought to keep their applicants guessing — that insecurity on the slave's part increases their ability to control. That couldn't be further from reality. Dominants who hide, deceive, or threaten in order to get what they want are probably not capable of entering into successful, satisfying M/s relationships.

Satisfaction

We probably don't give satisfaction the consideration it deserves. No one enters or stays in a relationship unless it satisfies. OK, many people seem to stay in apparently unsatisfactory relationships for many reasons, but that is no reason to ignore the need for mutually beneficial relationships. Applicants on both sides of the dynamic need to find ways and have the willingness to satisfy their partners and enjoy doing so. Of course, how each is satisfied may be entirely different, but that each one knows and enjoys the benefits of the relationship remains important.

Some might comment that it is the slave who must satisfy the master, as is certainly the case. Doing so, on the other hand, in no way diminishes the fact that the slave must experience satisfaction in the relationship as well. An unsatisfied slave will quickly find ways to end the relationship, even if ending it is a subconscious motive.

Since satisfaction is an internal feeling, only you can define what satisfies you. As you seek a partner, review your feelings about time spent with them, even if it's in a chat room or via e-mail. Does interacting with them make you feel good when it's over? Are you glad to have spent time sharing with them? Once you meet in real time, is that time well spent, enjoyable, and fulfilling? Remember you're doing this for your mutual satisfaction; so, be sure you get what you are seeking.

Empowerment

As is true of all healthy relationships, masters and their slaves help each to attain their goals, be they personal, career, financial, etc. It is certainly the duty of the master to lead his or her slave into the fullness of the slave's potential. What is less known, but just as important, is that it falls to the slave to empower his or her master to greatness as well.

For example, if you believe that I contribute anything to the BDSM community at large by my writing or my public speaking, let me remind you that I am empowered to do so by the service provided me: day in and day out, 24 hours a day, seven days a week, twelve months a year, by my faithful slave, Patrick.

His care for my health, home, and happiness leave me free to write, to travel, and to speak. I live, after all, as much off his income as mine. My health insurance is provided by his employer, not mine. I would be loathe to be away from home as much as I am, in service to kinky folks across the continent, if there weren't someone keeping the home fires burning, so to speak, until I return. Because of his attention to cooking, cleaning, laundering, and the like, I am free to do other things. I have no cares when it comes to a welcoming meal upon my return. When I leave, I know that the dirty clothes from the last trip will be clean and ready for my next one.

I have similar responsibilities. I must know my slave and know wherein lies his potential and help him achieve it. Over the years, for instance, I have challenged him to find a more satisfactory job. I have encouraged him to learn (and taught him some of it) web design. I have supported and applauded his desire to become active in one of our local leather clubs. For my part, he is free of the concerns of bill paying.

There is, of course, more to the master/slave relationship than I have written of here. You will find that there is caring, listening, loving, and sharing, just as in any other healthy relationship. Don't get so caught up in the kink of the relationship that you ignore the very important human sides that each of you share.

Complementary Qualities

Having discussed some of the qualities that masters and slaves share, I can now turn (albeit briefly) to those that are complementary — such as control and surrender, sadism and masochism, and initiative and response. These will also be covered more fully in later chapters.

Much like authority and obedience, the characteristics of control and surrender lend a practical dimension to the M/s relationship. In fact, the extent of control and the depth of surrender go far to express the quality of the relationship. Masters must be able to control themselves and exercise their control over their slave freely, though the means and extent of the actual control is a highly individualistic choice. Surrender, meanwhile, demonstrates the slave's trust and commitment to his or her master. Not unexpectedly, the degree of surrender determines a great deal in the M/s relationship. The fuller the surrender, the more intimate, exciting, and meaningful the relationship can be. Though surrender is the slave's gift, it behooves every master to encourage it, especially by being trustworthy.

We encourage surrender by letting it be known that we seek it, by noting it with gratitude, and by rewarding it. We also encourage it by our positive, caring, and accepting attitude of it and especially by never abusing it.

Many people assume that M/s relationships are sadomasochistic. That assumption is exactly the kind that one ought not to make, as SM need not be part of the M/s dynamic at all. Statistically (where's Mr. Gallup when you need him?), it is likely that SM does play a role between many, if not most, masters and their slaves. I'm just noting that it need not be so. If it is present, it is often an expression of control and surrender. It also may very simply be a fun way for the M/s couple to play.

We most likely think of initiative as being part of the master's role and that response belongs to the slave. In general, that is true, though we have to keep in mind that initiative on the part of the slave, when it is in tune with the master's desires, may be perfectly acceptable. Likewise, the master had better be responsive to the slave's needs, or the slave will look elsewhere to have those needs met. These topics will be further covered in the chapters to come.

Patrick Reflects: A Yin-Yang Sort of Thing

I've always admired the concepts of harmony and balance represented by the circular symbols of the yin and the yang in the way they reflect the dynamic of the master/slave relationship. At their best, master/slave relationships develop an interconnectedness that transcend the physical or emotional — a dance. They're about redefining your life because another exists. You breathe because they do. This doesn't happen overnight and you only recognize that it has become so after it has become a routine part of who you are. It's very much like the Chinese philosophy of interacting opposites, yin-yang, each of which has the seed of the other; each exists because the other does; each makes the other possible.

This comes about when what has driven you both to this relationship stems from the same expectations. We develop those long before we find a master, but often don't consider what they are until after the relationship has begun. While a relationship can overcome different expectations, doing so is not easy, and a healthy relationship can't exist if any of those involved feel cheated out of what they really wanted.

It is far better to explore your expectations beforehand so that you are more familiar with what they are. They can then act as a guide in your search. Because of the uniqueness of each relationship, expectations will vary and will change in importance as the relationship develops, but they have to be acknowledged before they can change.

I've seen it occur many times. A slave finds that things are not how he expected them to be. The way you are dominated makes it difficult to breathe. The authority is too strict or too lenient. Responsibility isn't taken or given. Trust seems to have unequal values. A sense of security is not there. You thought there'd be more bondage or you expected more of a social life than you have. A master/slave relationship won't be an egalitarian relationship, but it can be a fulfilling one if expectations are satisfied. Having a clear sense of your expectations will allow you to communicate them and have them addressed in positive and satisfying ways.

When I applied to be Sir's slave it was only after I had a clear sense of what I wanted out of the relationship. There were many things I didn't consider: I hadn't considered the possibility of other slaves being in the relationship or, for that matter, that my master would have a lover or a master of his own. I hadn't considered how public the relationship would be or how often visitors would come and go. All of these were things I faced early on. But I had considered what would be important to me, and when faced with these and other situations, I was easily able to adapt because the things I had held as important were also part of the experience.

We clicked right off, but this was, in part, because I had spent a lot of time preparing myself for this change in my life and also because Sir was somewhat of a known quantity to me. I'd read his book, *The Master's Manual,* and the columns he wrote for *Drummer* and *International Leatherman.* Having done so gave me clues to his style of dominance. His reputation in the leather community ensured a certain trustworthiness and responsibility.

Beyond the initial chemistry, we clearly enjoyed the fact that we were able to effectively communicate what we felt we wanted and this allowed us to quickly strip away the unimportant and work on those things about which we needed to reach agreement. Does it work this way for everyone? No, generally not, but the approach is sound and if you can keep from getting lost in the fantasy of slavery, you can focus on the things that will lay the foundation for a similar confidence.

Our lifestyle is a puzzle to outsiders. They don't understand what it is that makes it interesting and satisfying for us and it isn't necessary that they do. Ultimately, the people we can count on will move beyond the puzzle and tag it in a way with which they can deal. In any case, their acceptance is far more important than their understanding. This acceptance will come once they see the magic of your dance and the sense of fulfillment it brings to both of you.

After Reading Activities

Using your journal, write a 1,000 (or more) word essay describing your future life as a slave. What do you do? Where do you live? What do you say? What is required of you? How does it feel? Let your imagination go wild. Make sure you save what you have written for later.

Write your reflections on the questions found at the beginning of this chapter: How do I have to change to be what I want to become? How will you be different when you are a slave? What actions and decisions will, in fact, transform you from who you are now to what you seek to become?

Use your journal to write the names, e-mail addresses, and phone numbers of possible references. Contact them for permission to use them as such. Assure them of your discretion.

If you don't have any references, what can you do to create (find) them? Ask people at your next munch, club meeting, or party what they do about referencing. Use their answers to develop a list as to how you will develop references for yourself.

Pretend that you have received an e-mail from an applicant who says that he has felt betrayed by people he has met online and would like some assurances that you are a trustworthy person. Write a letter in your journal that you think will allay his fears by proving that you are trustworthy. Show it to a friend and ask for comments.

2

The Call To Serve

Virtue is the power of acting exclusively according to one's true nature. And the degree of virtue is the degree to which somebody is striving for and able to affirm his own being. [*]

One of the more difficult aspects of becoming a slave involves understanding the meaning, in terms of BDSM, of slavery itself. It is obvious that the definition found in most dictionaries is inadequate: "a person held in servitude as the chattel of another; a person who has lost control of himself and is dominated by something or someone." Chattel is defined as "an item of tangible movable or unmovable property except real estate, freehold, and the things which are parcel to it."

For this reason, as I previously discussed, what we in the BDSM community call slavery is actually the state of voluntary servitude. It may be seen, therefore, as having three primary characteristics. It is willed and involves obedience and service. Using those characteristics, then, let me define slavery as "the state in which a person chooses to be in a relationship of obedience and service to another."

I choose this definition for three reasons. First, slavery is a relationship and therefore, includes at least two people: the master and the slave. Second, it is important to emphasize the fact that the slavery is created by the will of the slave, the decision to submit and surrender to another, granting him or her control over one's self, who wills to accept such submission and surrender. Third, it is imperative that submission and surrender be manifested in real-time by obedience.

My definition is intentionally broad, since slavery can be, and often is, manifested in a wide variety of situations. The extent of control

[*] Tillich, Paul, *The Courage To Be*, Yale University Press, New Haven, 1952.

given and exercised, for instance, varies greatly. Some relationships are primarily sexual, while others may involve no sex whatsoever. Slavery may be limited by constraints of health, geography, time, finances, and family obligations, thereby giving them a wide range of manifestations. Indeed, the definition is meant to reflect my premise that, "All relationships are defined by the two people in them." Therefore, how the above definition actually applies to your master/slave relationship depends upon you and your partner. For that reason it is a negotiated and mutually agreed upon relationship.

As a relationship, a slave must be a slave to something or, more particularly in this case, to someone. For that reason, we need to be clear to speak of a slave as one who is both submitted and owned. As my mother used to say, "It takes two to tango." Those who desire slavery, but are not yet in an actual relationship, therefore, are best called slave wannabes, slave-applicants, slave trainees or slave apprentices.

One becomes a slave through a process of choosing to submit one's will to that of another. Since this book is about becoming a slave, the emphasis is on the slave's decision to submit. That being so in no way mitigates the fact that the master also chooses. I begin the discussion of choice, though, as coming from the submissive, since without the submissive's consent, there can be no slavery. Yes, the master must also consent, but I see the slave's offer of surrender and service first as a gift, received by the master.

Certainly, it behooves the master to set the scene, so to speak, for the slave to offer, but no amount of the master's attempt to convince or coerce is going to create the relationship. You can't, after all, force a "gift" from someone unwilling to bestow it. Would that we masters could simply kidnap those we wish to enslave — but that is a fantasy, the realization of which is illegal. Instead, we need to prove that we are worthy of the offer and show the slave-applicant that he has nothing to fear by making the offer and that he will find the result, his enslavement, well worth his "gift." As Patrick notes, "This is the essence of a successful M/s relationship."

Having consensually created the relationship, it must be made manifest in some kind of action — hence, the need for the master to exercise control and the slave to respond appropriately as an act of obedience. Being obedient is "submitting to the restraint or command of authority." It is manifest in action. In that regard, it is the doing of the master's will about which I will write more later.

Obedience is also an excellent sign of trustworthiness. An obedient slave earns a master's trust very quickly. Likewise on the master's part, performance of what he says he or she will do indicates that the master or mistress is trustworthy as well.

In my own negotiation with slave-applicants and the subsequent training that my slaves receive, I place great emphasis on obedience, since I see it as the simplest explanation of what it is that I am seeking. As I tell my slaves, "If you obey me, then I get everything else that I want."

The Purpose of Slavery

For those not familiar with a couple involved in a master/slave relationship, it can be quite difficult to imagine why a person would want to be someone's slave. Even those who are friends or acquaintances with a slave are often at a loss to understand the "why" of slavery. In fact, the why is often an elusive answer not easily arrived at, even by those in the relationship. Understanding the motivation to surrender and obey is a difficult problem, compounded by the fact that each individual has his or her own unique reasons for making such a choice. It is also difficult because slavery is easily and often seen as countercultural, precisely since we live in a "free" and democratic country based on the premise that "All men are created equal." We prize ourselves on being a country of peers, without class and distinction of rank, though both are, ironically and unfortunately, very prominent.

Still, slavery is a choice that one is free to make.

Why does one make that choice? As varied as the men and women who create M/s relationships, so too are the reasons for doing so. First among those, and almost universally agreed upon, is the sense of mission or destiny, that one was "born this way" or has what some refer to as a "slave heart." Becoming a slave, then, is simply doing what one perceives is best for them, most natural, and promising the greatest satisfaction in life. There is no rebuke to this calling. Those who know simply understand that this is how they were meant to be.

There are other reasons as well. As far as I can tell, the most powerful of these is the desire for empowerment. I see this as mutual empowerment and a responsibility that both the master and slave embrace as regards the other.

If the master is meant to control and hold responsibility for the slave, then it is easily seen that he or she is meant to do so in a way that empowers the slave to become that which is closest to the slave's highest potential. This may happen by giving support, advice, resources, encouragement, or instruction, enabling the slave to have the power to accomplish a given goal. As the master learns of the slave's talents and potential, he or she is in the unique place to encourage the slave to reach for that potential, and to lend resources and advice on how to realize it.

The same applies to the slave's empowerment of his master. By serving the master and thereby relieving him or her of a great many mundane chores, the slave frees the master to devote time and energy more fully to attaining their potential. Over the nine years he has served me, Patrick has been an invaluable partner in promoting my career, principally by his domestic and financial support of my endeavors, though he certainly has given me much encouragement, assistance, and advice as well. For one to be empowered in slavery the person must find one who is empowered by their submission.

Another acknowledged reason for becoming a slave is to be better able to participate in the power exchange called living. Because of the intimacy and deep trust that accrues to the master and the slave, the exchange of energy, however one might experience it, is greatly enhanced, thereby improving many other aspects of each individual's life. This, as with many of the reasons to become part of a master/slave coupling, is the same for all human relationships, be they economic, physical, intellectual, corporate, national, sexual, or marital.

As a human relationship, mastery and slavery is also based upon the myriad reasons that two or more people join together. It gives a sense of belonging, aids self-actualization, provides mutual support and protection, creates an increased opportunity for sexual activity, and is fun. In a very real sense, it unites the two as one.

For many, if not most, love is also a strong motivation — if not in the early stages of the relationship, certainly as the two bond more closely over time. Love is, after all, a prime motivation in the development of relationships. To think that love doesn't, won't, or can't be part of a master/slave relationship is foolhardy.

There are two fundamental aspects to consider when it comes to slavery. The first has to do with abstract slavery itself: a state to which one is drawn and in which one chooses to live. This aspect of the answer involves both an understanding of the general meaning and purpose of slavery and the realization that there is something within one's unique nature that draws them to this life.

It is obvious, though, that not everyone who is attracted to slavery in general is equally attracted to all masters. Therefore, there are very particular reasons for slavery that are unique to the couples themselves: namely, attributes such as attraction, devotion, and love. For this reason, many slaves struggle to find the master that both meets their definition of a master, and who is, in fact, the special master who will satisfy them. Masters have a similar challenge in that they must seek not only a slave, but specifically, a slave who meets their theoretical and practical requirements.

These dual considerations make an author's attempt to define and explain voluntary servitude more challenging. It is one thing for me to consider mastery and slavery in general, but quite another to discuss the very personal and particular way in which any given master and slave will live. Nevertheless, we can consider the general aspects of slavery: will, surrender, obedience, bonding, and service.

The Role of Will in a D/s Relationship

Consent rests as a foundation stone of our kinky communities. Will, of course, is integral to consent, since exercising our will is the heart of a consensual relationship — even one that lasts for the short period of a single scene. Will is defined in a variety of ways in my dictionary as: "Volition; Mental powers manifested as a wishing, choosing, desiring, intending;" and "A disposition to act according to principles or ends."

Slavery, therefore, has both a mental aspect (volition) and a physical one (manifestation). In that regard, we speak of an act of the will. In my mind they go together, to decide a thing and then to not act upon it is to decide again in favor of a different view. The adage, taught to me by a therapist a long time ago (I think that's where I picked it up) states it pretty clearly: "Not to decide is to decide."

In a real sense, mitigating circumstances, especially doubt, lack of data, and conflicting information, may appear to delay (and often do) a decision. Still, they are, in fact, forces that lead to the decision to postpone a decision or to make a different decision. For instance, the decision to go skiing may be delayed by the decision to wait until one knows how the skiing conditions will be.

That's why many masters set deadlines for those wanting to play with them. People who protest that they "can't decide" are, in fact, making decisions all the time. Deciding to delay a meeting, for instance, is an act of the will, a decision.

Another point is that slaves can, in fact, have strong wills. The idea that some choose slavery because of their inability to make decisions is obviously contradicted by the fact that they have decided to become a slave. Slaves certainly have volition. What sets them apart is that their wills are aligned with that of their master.

That stated, there are numerous ways to consider the use of one's will in a M/s relationship: in terms of negotiation, as an empowering force that brings us to a certain depth, edge, or experience, as an act that unites and binds us together psychologically and intellectually, leading to other forms of bonding as well. Whereas there is some talk about "breaking one's will," I prefer to see this breaking, not as destructive *per se*, but as preparatory to a realignment of wills.

Negotiations are the means we use to gather enough information to make an informed decision as to how, when, and with whom we will play, both in terms of a simple scene or as regards a long-term relationship

(LTR). Here, the words "I can't decide" are simply a euphemism. We can always decide. Our ability to exercise our intellect and emotions themselves is seldom impaired. That doesn't mean that we can always make a good decision. The words "I can't decide" usually indicate that one does not have enough information to make what one would think is a good decision. Rather than say, "I can't decide," one ought to say, "I don't have enough information to make a decision that I would find satisfactory," thereby recognizing the need for further negotiation.

My observation is that bottoms have more difficulty with the decision-making process than tops, though that may be merely an expression of my own rather decisive nature. Still, there is a tendency among bottoms, and especially those who believe they ought to be more submissive, that to utter a decision is somehow unacceptable. I can only guess why this might be the case, but I can venture that one might think that appearing decisive indicates the lack of a submissive nature. I would argue to the contrary.

First off, we are always making decisions, even if we simply call them preferences, choices, or doing what we are told. When, for instance, Patrick asks me "What do you want for breakfast, Sir?" the answer "I don't care," is not helpful at all, unless you read in it the decision that "Whatever you serve will be satisfactory." Of course, that's not true, since if he served me fried pig brains for breakfast, I would have reason to rue my inability or unwillingness to name a more desirable meal.

Secondly, I am not willing to spend my whole life micromanaging a bottom's life by deciding for him. Even if I were wont to do so, in order for me to state what their will should be, I would have to know a great deal about their preferences, prejudices, limits, and experiences. I grant that I could possibly (but not probably) make every decision needed to live Patrick's life. After all, his will is rather well aligned with mine and after nine years, I know him rather well. Still, I'm not about to decide if he should walk to the "El" stop or take the bus, if he should check for messages on the answering machine before or after he checks his e-mail, or whether he has to urinate or not. Give me a break. I have a life and so does he.

In the intensity of a given scene is where we can most easily see the effect of will, since not only does it often involve an *a priori* decision ("OK, single tail me until I am bleeding."), it also involves the use of the will in continuing what one's body might scream to end. ("I'm OK. Please don't stop," he said as the whip made his back bleed.) Here we see the power of the mind over the body most forcefully. We agree to let the decision stand, even when our bodies act to make it cease. In fact, we very often use bondage in just such a scene in order to help the mind control the screaming and squirming physical aspect of our bodies.

Often, too, one of the important and real victories for many in SM is the sense of accomplishment earned when the will does control the actions of the body. In a very real sense, it is a triumph of the mind over the body and usually one which the body comes to enjoy as well, despite demonstrations to the contrary.

One further point about will is that we need to differentiate it from wishing and fantasy. For many, slavery will never become a reality because they will never decide to make it such. Instead they use the seeking of a master (usually online) as a way to satisfy their erotic life without making the necessary commitment to obedience, devotion, and surrender of their will. Patrick says that wannabes such as these are "playing a good game, but have no intention of following through to a real level. Their game improves with practice, improving their online erotic life, while negating any need to make one's slavery real."

The third area we can consider is the "breaking of one's will." Mirroring the drama of enforced slavery, such as in prisons, concentration camps, and torture scenarios, some think that form of slavery must be imposed; the slave's will needs be obliterated, creating a robot to the master's whims. As noted above, I don't think this is either a necessary or desirable action. What is desirable is the removal of impediments to the unity of wills. Yes, I may beat a man into submission. The beating, though, is meant to bring pleasure, to show the slave that surrender to the whip, for instance, will bring real joy. Experiencing my whip in such a way gives him an incentive to surrender to me for the purpose of experiencing the joy of that surrender.

Having said — at least by implication — "Sir, I am yours," he can then begin to internalize the meaning of that which he was (agreeably) forced to utter; it is hoped that eventually, this will make the words true. The end result is not a broken will, but rather one conformed to the will of the one dominating him. It is this alignment of wills that creates a deeper and more lasting bond between top and bottom, master and slave. The desired (or should I write "willed") effect, then, is that in a practical sense, there is only one will: that of the dominant — though in truth, the submissive will continually be called upon to realign his or her will to that of the dom(me).

Granted, there are certainly times when the expression of one's will is pronounced, such as when a master and slave reach agreement on entering the relationship or when they celebrate their mutual commitment with a collaring ceremony. In actuality, both are called upon to reaffirm their decisions to be so related on a daily, if subconscious, level.

Surrender

One of the more important qualities in creating fulfilling relationships, in general — and the master/slave relationship, in particular — is the partners' abilities to surrender to one another and to the relationship. When this happens, incredible experiences become possible, if not probable. Surrender offers the slave a real sense of freedom, of release, and of bonding with the one to whom he or she surrenders. In moments of intense surrender, there are real feelings of security, peace, and bliss.

The slave's surrender increases the master's sense of control and his ability to dominate. The master's surrender to mastery allows him or her to experience a deeper and more meaningful actualization of that mastery.

Before we can surrender, though, certain requirements must be met concerning safety, responsibility and trust. Please keep those conditions in mind as you read this section, since without trust and the assurance of mutual safety, surrender becomes a bad, if not dangerous, idea. In every case, then, one ought to read the word surrender with the clear understanding that we are talking about responsible surrender, not irrational abandonment or insane escapism.

Responsible surrender recognizes that there are physical, emotional, legal, and spiritual limits that define one's surrender. It is surrender that includes the necessary, but mundane, chores of life, that realizes that our humanity remains an important part of who we are, that understands that the best decisions and actions are based on a holistic approach that includes the whole self.

True slavery includes meeting the financial, social, and familial responsibilities that one has to oneself and one's family. Those who seek slavery as a way to avoid child support, escape from a less than satisfying relationship, or because they prefer daily bondage in the basement to a nine-to-five job, are being irresponsible.

According to my handy dictionary, surrender is: "to relinquish possession or control of to another because of demand or compulsion; to give up in favor of another." Since compulsion is obviously not part of healthy BDSM, we might amend the definition to: "relinquish possession or control of in favor of another." We do so for the benefits that such surrender will give us.

On the other hand, compulsion can certainly come from within. The submissive understands that slavery is his best course in life, that true happiness will come from surrendering, and nothing less than true surrender will ever be satisfying.

It is natural to see this in the master/slave dynamic, but it applies, in some degree, to all our activities. Likewise, we might assume that surrender only applies to the bottom when, in fact, it applies to both players. In that regard, we are looking at either mutual surrender or surrender to a third entity or quality. It can be seen that slaves are to surrender to their masters. In a similar vein, masters are required to surrender to their mastery. Even the sex masters need to surrender to the act and in some ways, surrender to their partners.

Here, I am at a loss for words. As a top, I sometimes experience the desire to surrender to my own passion, lusts, and desires. As an example, occasionally when mounting Patrick from behind I have experienced strong desires to bite and scratch him, accompanied by a desire to growl and roar. I am overcome, at times, with the feeling of being a lion. At other times, I feel like an eagle. Surrendering to these feelings and allowing myself to undergo these psychological (and short-lived) changes, intensifies the encounter. To do so, though, takes a certain amount of surrender of self to the fantasy of being a lion or an eagle.

It is not an uncommon event. There is a point, fleeting as it may be, in every act of orgasm where one surrenders to his or her sexual passion and the natural course of events transpires. For men, when the penis decides to shoot, there can often be no stopping it, though with practice it is possible. Why else do we joke that a penis has a "head of its own"?

I start with this line of thinking to ensure that we see surrender as part and parcel of good sex for both (all) partners. It would be easy to stipulate that surrender applies to the bottom, as the activities look that way to an observer. But looks can be deceiving and there can be lots of BDSM and/or sex that contains little or no surrender.

My point is that between trusting, committed, and experienced partners, surrender becomes both an issue and a way to deepen (or is it heighten?) both the experience and the relationship. It should be obvious that we are not talking here about casual SM, tricks, or quick sex. Those activities are places where some of us start, but in time, most of us come to feel a need for a better quality to our sex, and surrender is one of the ingredients that brings us there.

Because surrender makes one vulnerable, I began this section with a paragraph about trust, safety, and responsibility. Surrender is no easy feat. In order to surrender, we must know that to whom or what we surrender will not injure us in any way.

Early on, for instance, in my slavery to Master Lynn, I realized that to gain the full potential of my slavery, I had to allow him to play with me as he willed. Fortunately, it was easy for me to find reason to trust him. I, therefore, had to accept my own masochistic side, surrendering to his sadistic nature. I had to give up some of my decision making prerogatives, especially when I was in his home or he in mine. I had to surrender control over things such as my ability to have an orgasm, my choice of restaurants, the schedule of my weekend.

In SM and sexual play, there is often the need to surrender to one's partner, allowing that person the right to do things that might be otherwise unacceptable. I think here of the master's playing with the slave's rectum or putting his fingers in the slave's mouth. I hope you wouldn't let just anyone do that to you. What is inappropriate for a stranger on the commuter train, may be the master's prerogative. The slave, then, regardless of his desires concerning such activity, grants the master the power to enjoy that which he desires. In this case, it is paramount that the slave's focus be on the master's pleasure, rather than on his own.

Healthy relationships are those that are able to grow. Stagnant relationships are bound to be in trouble, sooner or later. Increased surrender is one way to move a relationship into greater depth and intensity. I think that's one of the ways that Patrick and I have been able to keep so much fun in our master/slave relationship: I have continually, albeit slowly, demanded more surrender, more slavery from him, and have accepted more responsibility, more mastery on my part. The result is that play, which would have been unimaginable nine years ago, is now rather easily accomplished.

Our long-term relationship has given rise to a deep level of trust, allowing each of us to surrender, as necessary. That surrender allows us to intensify our play and to remove limits that seemed immoveable earlier in the relationship. Surrender allows for an ever-expanding repertoire of physical and emotional enjoyment.

The idea for this topic arose out of my consideration of surrender during sex. Considering it more holistically is important as well. What happens (or doesn't) in the bedroom is very much determined by your relationship outside the bedroom. This leads us to ask: "How can an increase in surrender in other areas of our relationship open us to greater bonding, deeper intimacy, and a healthier relationship in general?" Better sex is a good motive, but there is much more to sex than simply the sex act.

Of course, that line of thinking brings me once again to the necessity for the partners to communicate well. It is too easy to look at our relationships superficially, to think that surrender is a quick and easy solution, without any consideration of what it means.

For slaves, surrender is what allows them to realize the fullness of their desires, their need for slavery. As they become more surrendered, they become more slavish and therefore, more closely realize their true nature. In that sense, the slave's surrender is actually as critical to their authentic selves as to anyone or anything.

As we begin to surrender one to another, problems can be seen simply as signals that there are questions to be asked, motives to be sought, and solutions to be found. The surrender we seek, after all, has to come from all of our being. It is not just an intellectual exercise or something we do only with our genitalia.

Genuine surrender demands commitment, understanding, and the willingness to bare oneself as completely as possible. That means that the one to whom we surrender must be trustworthy, responsible, and that he or she not abuse the very sacred trust we are giving them. All of this, of course, takes time. This is why real surrender comes not in the moment, but in the long-term. It is not taken for granted, but given because it is earned.

Obedience

If I seem to harp on the idea of obedience, it is because I refuse to see slavery as a fantasy, a charade, or merely an intellectual or semantic exercise. It is a relationship and one which is best manifested by the slave's obedience to the master's will and direction.

There are, of course, some who enjoy the scenario of a rebellious slave. I would not call this mastery and slavery. For me, it is best categorized as role-playing, an often highly-erotic and pleasant pastime, but hardly one of control and obedience. It may be completely satisfactory theater or sexually fulfilling play, but it is not the essence of a long-term relationship.

To obey means: "To carry out or fulfill the command, order, or instruction of." Obedience then, is seen as the effect of the master's will exercised by the slave who fulfills that will. If a slave doesn't behave as commanded, what is the sense of calling the relationship one of mastery and slavery?

There certainly are limits and qualifications to obedience. If there is no change (i.e., if that which is commanded is not done), then there is no obedience. Intentions are all well and good, but action is what makes the relationship real.

Clarifying the qualifications to obedience is needed. What is commanded must be done so clearly. Otherwise, how can the slave perform that which he or she either doesn't know or understand? If the directions are unclear, it falls upon the submissive to ask for clarity and for the dominant to ensure that such clarity is present. A good rule of management is for the master to take responsibility to guarantee that commands are understood.

Obedience, too, may be of a more general nature rather than in the giving of direct commands. Patrick, for instance, isn't told to cook dinner every night or when to do the laundry. He knows that he is responsible for the running of the household and does so without my direct intervention. Dinner appears, clean clothes are where they should be, and the bathroom gets cleaned. I am happy and served, even if I haven't spent my life commanding his every minute.

Since the slavery is negotiated, there may also be a *priori* limits to the slave's requirement to obey. Certainly, there are physical, legal, moral, and emotional limits to what the slave can do. Here, it becomes the responsibility of each to make certain that the orders do not violate the spirit or letter of the agreement between master and slave.

Certainly, you can find endless debate about the place of obedience in the life of the slave. Obedience is circumscribed by possibility, by the limits of time, place, talent, and available resources. Legal and other requirements also dictate certain limits to obedience as well.

It is important, then, to consider the reality (even if you both choose to do otherwise) that obedience is limited (or ought to be) by responsibility. There are those who say otherwise, believing that the slave's obligation is to obey the master without qualification. I will leave the balance between obedience and responsibility to the individuals in the relationship, who will then have to live with the consequences of their decisions.

Time clarifies obedience. Just as a slave learns the patterns of the master's expectations, so too do masters learn the difference between a slave's disobedience and his misunderstanding of an order.

Bonding

As master and slave enter into and deepen their relationship, we find that bonding is one of slavery's purposes. The interaction of master and slave, the surrender of the one to the will of the other, creates an intense and highly satisfactory bond: "A uniting force," between both members of the relationship. This bond is, in itself, highly pleasurable and fulfills strong and essential humans needs of belonging, of purpose, and of experiencing a real sense of wholeness.

Bonding is what often sustains the other elements of the relationship. It gives added rationale to the service, the sex, the trust, and the obedience. At times, bonding can even be the stronger element in the relationship, holding it together when other characteristics may be temporarily weakened. It can be an important "cement" that keeps master and slave together when they experience the usual downs of daily living.

For this reason, as the relationship develops, we often find affection, camaraderie, and tenderness deepening in the relationship. Though they may not have been seen as original purposes, such rationales often develop because of the close bonding that occurs.

Service

As a purpose for slavery, two dynamics shape service: The master takes on a slave in order to be served. The slave has discerned an inner desire or need to be of service — that is: "To work for; to be of assistance to or promote the interests of; aid."

Service itself can bring its own rewards. There is satisfaction in a job well done. There is pleasure in knowing that one has contributed to the success of another. There is fulfillment in the heart of one who believes that he is meant to serve.

One can see the reality of this in the lives of slaves who are proud of their masters' successes and who relish the praise given their masters, knowing full well that it is their service that has made such praise possible. Indeed, my readers know — as I have written more than once — that my slave, Patrick, must be credited for his role in my writing. After all, if I had to work as hard in the house as he does, this book would certainly have taken a lot longer to write.

The Call Itself

The most powerful rationale for entering into voluntary servitude is that the slave experiences an inner need or desire to do so. Akin to the inner "call" to a religious vocation, slavery originates in the "heart" of one who is called.

Here, of course, it is difficult to give precise language as to how this call is perceived. For some, it arises spontaneously. For others, it is ever-present from one's earliest memories. For still others, the idea to become a slave is spawned by a novel, a magazine, or a movie, beginning as the germ of an idea and evolving into a firm resolution that such a lifestyle is going to bring the most fulfillment and satisfaction to one's life. For some, slavery is simply inspired by the dominant.

There are those, too, for whom the "call" seems to have always been there. Many who fall into this category choose service-oriented careers, such as nursing or the ministry, to later find that their need to serve is more encompassing. When they discover the possibility of having a master and slave relationship, they easily respond to it.

Indeed, even the word "call" provides dubious insight: "To summon to a particular career or pursuit," since we are at a loss to understand who or what does the calling and how it is actually experienced. What can be said is that the call is unique to the person "hearing" it. For some, it begins as a fantasy, for others by seeing the life of another slave or as a presentation at a BDSM event. As one explores the possibility of actualizing it, the idea of slavery takes on a life of its own, becoming an incessant and highly attractive alternative to be lived for the rest of one's life. In that regard, the call is usually one that grows. Its meaning becomes refined by research and experience, until one has an inner assurance that a life of committed surrender, obedience, and service is that which most closely satisfies the mysterious, inner voice called soul, conscience, or heart.

Patrick Reflects: Answering the "Call"

I've never been quite comfortable with phrases like "call to slavery or service," or "slave heart." The former seems to suggest the possibility of not really having a choice in the matter, while the latter seems to take away the responsibility of making a choice. Voluntary servitude is all about choosing, and if you are offering more than that, you are probably offering more than you have to give.

For me, it isn't a call to serve, perhaps because I was convinced once before that I was called (to the ministry) and never felt it was where I was supposed to be. Though I was productive and successful, I wasn't fulfilled and was never comfortable in the role. I doubt that the call I felt sitting in that church pew was calling me to slavery (though some will say there are certainly some parallels). I'd convinced myself of something, but it certainly didn't fit right.

No, it isn't a call. It's much better than that.

Eroticism is at the heart of who we are as kinky folks. When I discovered it was okay to be erotic, it opened ways of being that I couldn't give a name to before, other than to feel it as fear. We are at our best when we are in tune with the erotic side of our nature. It frees us to be so much more than we would be without that freedom.

I serve because it makes me "hard" deep down. My cock might or might not show it, but deeply within myself, service is sexy and fulfilling. That combination is both powerful and life changing.

It's only when you've finally tapped into that place that you realize that doing so is very natural. Peel away everything else and it's all about being sexual and sex is as pure as it gets, folks. I think anyone who tries to wrap service in seemingly loftier garb is merely wrapping it in a fig leaf, trying to hide the power that it has. Slave service loses its meaning and magic when it quits being erotic.

My slavery does contain some altruism, but it has to contain much more than that to keep me choosing to serve.

That's where the meaning began for me, though I didn't really understand it when I first discovered voluntary servitude in a magazine in an adult bookstore. Service can be very erotic. I guess you could say that the artist Brick was the apostle who brought the message to me in

46

the way he captured it all in his sketch in Issue 32 of *Drummer*.[†]

It wasn't a calling I was answering. It was a longing to be who I really was.

After Reading Activities

Take some time to consider what it is that you want and why you want it. You might use your journal to express this answer or ask a friend or mentor to explore the answer with you.

What kind of decisions are you willing to make about becoming and/or being a slave? What reasons prompt you to do so? What things make you hesitate? What are the doubts that you feel? What keeps you from deciding?

Are you ready and able to surrender, given the right conditions? What are those conditions? How have you experienced surrender, either on the giving or the receiving end?

What factors in your everyday life obstruct your ability to surrender or to make a commitment? How can you reduce or eliminate these barriers to developing an M/s relationship.

Answer these questions in your journal, or bring the questions to a discussion group and explore them there.

[†] See Appendix D.

3

Finding a Partner

We must be our own before we can be another's.[*]

It is difficult to know where to start when one gives advice on finding a partner, even for an author who's trying to write a book about it. As I hope you've figured out by now, slavery involves a master. Therefore, successful slavery means that you end up in a real-time relationship.

What may be less easy to figure out is that the process begins by knowing oneself. That, of course, is really a never ending, lifelong task; while we learn who we are, we continually change and grow into being someone else.

This self-knowledge, as far as voluntary servitude is concerned, begins with that quiet call described in the last chapter. Sadly, there won't be much more detail than what's there. That is because the call involves a highly individualized and personal voice; it comes in a wide variety of ways, at different times, and for a great number of reasons.

Further complicating the idea of a call is that the call is generally progressive, even evolutionary. It is a call that grows with its being heard and acted upon, clarified by reflection and experience. It is my hope that by the time you finish this book, you will know whether your call is real or not and have found the courage to follow it to your heart's content.

If you are unsure about knowing yourself, my advice is that you find some good books or a mentor who can lead you to a better understanding of the process, since in itself it is a whole other book.

---

[*]   Emerson, Ralph Waldo, *Friendship Essays*, First Series, 1841.

Your Unique Expression

Despite myths to the contrary, slavery is the unique expression of that which both you and your master bring to the relationship. I know you'd all love to have exact rules and regulations for some cookie-cutter coupling, but such does not exist. Each of the couples who have shared their experiences with me made it clear that their lives are wonderfully and wholly their own. None would recommend copying what they do. In fact, most masters began their interview with me with the same caution, "Jack, I'm the only one who does it this way."

What they were saying is that what each master/slave couple has in common is their ability to be themselves, making them different from all the others. So then, in a real sense, the definitions by which you live will be your own. Thankfully, there are some guidelines. You have seen many of them in the opening chapters of this book. They can serve as goals and guideposts to creating a healthy and satisfying M/s relationship. Certainly, there are more in the following chapters.

The idea of slavery has two parts: the general meaning and living of a D/s relationship, and the refinement that each partner brings to the relationship based upon his or her own values, tastes, and choices.

This knowing what slavery is, and knowing what it is for you and your partner, is an ongoing process. In a way, it can seen as circular: we begin with an idea of slavery and explore that meaning. Our exploration, such as through reading or attending a seminar, brings us more knowledge that refines and expands the first definition. We might, then, have some kind of experience with slavery which brings further clarity to the definition.

Having come thus far, our own reflection on the experience, and our response (reaction) to it, then adds a further dimension from which we can continue exploration, research, and experimentation, arriving once again at reflection. This process continues until we have found that one definition that best fits us. That is not to say that the defining is done, nor that there is nothing left to learn. Instead, we have arrived at some basis for a meaningful search for the "other" who sees his or her mastery in a light which is complementary to our vision of slavery.

For better or for worse, most slave wannabes simply post an ad and hope for the best, without a clear idea of what that might mean. Unfortunately, they fail to define what they want and have no strategy for getting it, other than waiting. Like any other career, slavery does, indeed, have a natural educational path; becoming a slave entails a great deal more than simply wishing. Becoming a slave is an active, not a passive, process.

Knowing yourself and what you want is the difficult part of the process and really ought to be addressed before you start your search. Once this all important question is answered, the fundamental requirement for finding a partner is action.

Fantasy is pleasurable, especially when one is masturbating, but no amount of dreaming will make your partner appear unless effort is added to idea. I wish I could tell you that effort by itself is sufficient, but it is not. What is required is informed, patient, and persevering effort. Remember that you have to "Kiss a lot of frogs to find a prince."

There are no statistics available as to what constitutes "a lot of frogs." It is my experience that the quantity is probably more than 500. Responses to ads and e-mails are a dime a dozen — or less — as the initial response rate is liable to be very high, with a success rate that seems miniscule. After all, one in five hundred is only two-tenths of one percent. On the other hand, finding one master or one slave will most likely make the 499 failures seem well worth it.

That's why I added the adjectives patient and persevering to the word effort. Your search will be a roller coaster of hopes raised and dashed. The best advice on the subject came from a national sales manager I once worked with, who told me, "Just remember that every no brings you one no closer to yes."

Those noes increase the statistical chances that you will get to a yes, but there is another reason that the advice is good advice. Each no contains a lesson as to what you have to do differently, if your search is to be informed. "Keep on doing what you've always done and you will keep on getting what you've always gotten." Therefore, change in the process of searching is both inevitable and necessary. No increases the likelihood of success because it holds some clue as to how you can continue your search more effectively.

Analyze your "failures" to see what you might have done differently. Ask someone with expertise to look at them with you, as someone else's eyes are going to be a great deal more objective, hence more accurate, than yours.

I found my slave, Patrick, for instance, after my friend Bobby volunteered to rewrite my classified ad. What he produced was entirely different, though completely factual, to the one I had been running. His most significant change was the inclusion of the word "Ready." Up until that time I had obviously attracted many men, none of whom were ready for the changes necessary to becoming my slave. Being ready means a great variety of things which can best be perceived by the one who wants to be partnered. One applicant, for example, thought he was ready, but when faced with the rigorous social life of his potential master, found that his health was not up to the relationship. A year and a half later, his health having been restored to a higher level of vigor, he recontacted the master.

Other determining factors may be family obligations. You would be amazed by how many closeted married men want to desert their wives and children to become slaves. Likewise, married couples might have to tailor or curtail their D/s or M/s relationships in light of live-at-home children or careers.

Debt, too, is a handicap to mastery and slavery. Slavery alone rarely delivers an applicant from financial worries. One of my interviewees was a master who took control of his slave's income, eliminating the slave's debt over time; he used the slave's money, not his own, but this is probably the exception that proves the rule.

One of the most frequent comments I receive about finding the right person is, "There are no masters (or slaves) where I live." Those who so inform me invariably live in large cities. I've heard that lament about Los Angeles, San Francisco, Chicago, and New York — and I live in Chicago!

What the whining applicants are really saying is that they're not looking in the right way. Most often, it seems to me, that is because they don't want their friends to know they're looking. That is unfortunate, since friends can be a valuable connection to other applicants — if your friends are scene-friendly. For that reason, I can't say too strongly that sincere applicants should be active in the D/s scene where they live.

Being so offers a great number of benefits. First, that's where the other applicants are probably looking as well. Second, the local scene can offer you a place to find a mentor and advice. Third, it's far easier to meet someone from across town, and certainly a lot less expensive, than it is to do so across the country.

Expectations

A man named Randy, who was seeking a master, once posted a question about expectations on a newsgroup; he wanted to know what masters expected from applicants. Among his suggested answers were: "The usual, obedience, respect, control, dominance, service and excellent communications and so on."[†] My initial reaction was that we masters ought to have no expectations, but that remark probably only reflects my jaded opinion.

More to the truth, we all have expectations. I would say, though, that the ones suggested above are extremely premature, just as my having no expectations is probably false. If anything, I expect rejection, incompetence, and a gross lack of manners.

Reality surely exists somewhere between the two. Let me take the

---

† Slave boy, Randy, posted this question on March 18, 2004 to REALMastersNslaves, a Yahoo group.

lack of expectations first.

It's not true that I have no expectations. Rather, my expectations are limited, due to the great number of disappointing applications I have received. As an example, I have received some thirty-seven e-mails from a guy in Chicago who wants me to train him as a slave. He repeatedly says he'll call or come over, but never does. Hey, I can take a hint. This guy is a loser, afraid of his own shadow. I can quote experiences like that over and over. In the past four years, I have received over 1,600 messages from guys (and a few gals) seeking to become my slave. That averages more than one a day, from which I think I can safely say I've met about six people. Now, that's not 1,600 people who have written — but it is probably more than 300. Statistics such as these tend to reduce one's expectations.

So, now I only expect a reply. Well, to be closer to the truth, I hope for a reply. Since most applicants don't get past the second reply, I no longer expect much.

My "timetable for enthrallment" outlines my expectations once I know that I can expect something. So, I expect you to communicate with me for about a month, asking questions and answering mine. If we are still communicating then, I will invite you to meet me, either at my place or at an event. If you're local, I only expect to meet and say so, without any promise of sex or anything else. If you are traveling (I expect at your own expense), then I will offer you the hospitality of my home, with the proviso that you can switch from slave-applicant to tourist if, in the course of our meeting, that seems like a good idea. If you agree to a visit, my expectations will begin to rise. On the other hand, I have had numerous cancellations of the negotiations at this point, as words are significantly cheaper than airplane tickets.

Expectations grow as trust in each other is earned. That is why I think that Randy's expectations are unrealistic. He doesn't say at what level of intimacy his expectations are expected. To think that a complete stranger is going to obey, control, dominate, serve, or even communicate excellently is beyond my imagination. To Randy's credit, there are a lot of master-applicants who indeed might have those expectations, but they are unrealistic and without foundation.

As I wrote earlier, obedience must come from authority and the master-applicant certainly has no authority over a slave-applicant he's never met. Trust must be earned and isn't earned easily. Most people are terrible communicators. They can talk well enough, but listening, probing, and clarifying are rare arts. It is as simple as that.

Rather than expectations, I think it is more correct to see the process, from initial contact to long-term relationship, as one of mutual testing. Randy's question might better be "What do masters test in their applicants?" Whether they admit to it or not, slave-applicants are testing the suitability of their master-applicants as well.

First off, both master and slave must be realistic as they begin the dialogue. Neither is superior (nor inferior) to the other. Both are free adults, entitled to courtesy and respect. While both might be trustworthy, each has to earn the other's trust. Though both may be competent, that competency must be proven by action. Assumptions are odious and dangerous. To assume, after all, makes an ass of u and me. So, we do this little dance, trying to ascertain whether the other is trustworthy. We are looking for sincerity, honesty, and openness.

I know that ads are replete with other criteria: age, weight, skin color, HIV status, employability, you name it. In truth, all these criteria only make the search more difficult. Is there, after all, much difference between a 35 year old and one who is 36? In any case, if your successful 29 year old applicant actually becomes your slave, in due time he'll be over forty. Are you going to kick him out when he reaches some "too old" birthday? What if your lean muscle machine gains 50 pounds, does that end the relationship?

It is important for the master to communicate as fully as possible. It is necessary for the slave-applicant to make sure that he or she understands what is being said. If I haven't made it clear, let me state in no uncertain terms: Both master and slave are applicants. For a successful relationship to develop, each one must freely choose the other.

Yes, sometimes I get tired of applying to become someone's master. I know that many slave-applicants get weary with the process as well. How many frogs do you have to kiss to find a prince?

So, I watch what my newest applicant does. Does he ask questions? Does he seem to answer honestly? When I ask him to do something, does it get done?

The high number of applicants who can't call when they say they will, don't answer simple e-mails, or fail to obey the simplest request, would amaze you. By not responding appropriately, they effectively cut themselves out of the process. This is unfortunate because it means that neither of us gets nearer to our objective: ownership.

I think that one of the reasons that this happens so frequently is that we have false expectations about the interview process. Slaves think that the master is in charge; in actuality, both are responsible. I'm thinking, for instance, of those men who read an e-mail; then, reading into it more than they should, stopped the correspondence, thinking, "I could never do that."

That doubt is based on an expectation of going from free individual to complete slave in one great leap. In fact, the "jump right in" fantasy is unrealistic. Ditch it. It will never happen. OK, I shouldn't use never;

so, I'll just say that it seldom happens. What does happen is that there is (and needs to be) a long process of getting to know one another, gaining and earning trust, until each knows that they are both suited to this relationship.

Even at that point, there will most likely be a long, slow process until the final result is met. There'll be visits, and numerous phone calls, and e-mails. Short weekend visits will turn into spending a week together, then longer, until the slave is collared and plans are set for living in a long-term relationship.

Early Protocols

Despite my foul opinion of expectations, because many in the M/s community do have them, I would be remiss not to mention some expected protocols.

Masters usually like to be called "Sir." Some, of course, don't. The best advice about this is to simply ask your master-applicant politely: "Would you please tell me what your preferred title is at this point in our conversation?" Once you find out, by all means use it. Masters have a reciprocal responsibility: Know what you want to be called and when. I'm probably in the minority when I say I want to be called Jack. Only after the dialogue proves there is some real interest will I then request that I be called Sir.

You both should have some idea of how quickly you want to proceed. Unfortunately, you will find that there are a great number of dreamers out there who are simply looking out of curiosity or unrequited lust. Be real in your search, and be realistic in what you can do and how soon you can do it. If there are limits to your making a move now, make them clear to your applicants. There's nothing wrong in settling for a part-time or short-term relationship, if that is what is necessary, but be honest about that from the beginning.

Be prompt to answer e-mails and return phone calls, even if it's to say that you're too busy to answer, but that there will be a response in such and such a time frame. I can't be too emphatic about this. Keep in contact with your prospective masters or slaves, if only to send a quick greeting.

Slave-applicants can expect to pay for their first trip to visit prospective owners. After that, you can probably expect to share costs, depending upon individual circumstances.

You both should have an idea of what you want to know and what you think your applicant should know early on. I have gotten into the habit, for instance, of asking a set of easy questions quite soon; that allows me to gauge whether the applicant is at least a possibility. I also inform them of possible negatives about myself — sooner rather than later. In other words, I would rather get disqualified now and move on, than waste lots of time and energy on interviews that will go nowhere. Applicants who hide the truth are going to get outed eventually. If you're older, overweight, or have some impediments, it really is best to get those facts on the table now, not later.

Since a picture is usually expected, have a few made. You can copy them on a copier to save the expense of prints or scan them as j-pegs. They need not be nude shots, though many people like that. The exposed body pictures can be sent when there is a higher level of trust that they won't be posted on the Internet. Don't laugh. I know applicants who have sent phony pictures. One guy even got his own photo back from an applicant.

Yes, you can expect early questions about what kind of kink you like. You will also be asked about what you have to offer the successful candidate. Have, then, a few ready answers and be willing to explain why.

A last suggestion is that you take care to use a spell-checker, look over your grammar, and remember that neatness counts. A good piece of advice is to print out any written material and read out loud to yourself before you send it off. Have a friend look it over, if possible, since you'll want to avoid sending material that contains errors.

The Search

Before you begin your search, it's important that you know what you want to find. That's why I had you do the imagination exercise at the end of chapter two.[‡] I hope by now that you know what your criteria are.

If you've not done that, then it needs be on your to do list. You wouldn't believe how many applicants don't know what they want. They have no answer when asked, "What do you mean when you say you want to be a slave?"

I'm still waiting for a friend, who wants to be a master, to tell me what kind of slave he wants. When I posed the question, he admitted he didn't know and that he would get back to me. A year later, he still hasn't answered the question.

I cannot stress too strenuously that one needs to be careful about "what you want to find." The more specific your criteria, the more difficult it's going to be to find that special someone. It is as basic as that. A broader definition, after all, includes more possibilities.

You will find, too, that the longer you search, the fewer will be the number of requirements you have, as the search itself will force reality upon your thinking. Quite frankly, limiting candidates by age,

‡   It's not too late to go back and do it now.

geography, physique, education, or any other number of criteria often proves futile. You are much better off to cast a wider net than a smaller one.

History proves, too, that in a great many cases, successful couples found partners who hardly matched the men or women they originally sought. When, therefore, you demand that your applicant have certain qualifications, you may be eliminating just the applicant who will make the best master or slave for you. The more open you are to possibilities, the higher will be your probabilities. It is as straightforward as that.

The Ad

For most of us, the quest for a partner leads to a personal ad. In years past, they were mostly found in the back of magazines or newspapers. Those ads were a substantial part of the publisher's revenue. That was generated either from the prices charged to run the ad, or from the "postage and handling fee," usually a dollar per ad — charged to the one sending an answer to a blind post office box. The response was then forwarded to the person placing the ad, if such a person existed. In some instances, the ad had been placed by the publisher, looking to earn a few extra dollars.

Response rates to ads have always been dismal, but even dismal is slightly better than none at all. So, the ads eventually lead to a meeting.

It's important to note that placing and responding to ads is virtually a numbers game. The odds increase only slightly by writing a better ad.

In recent years, the personals have almost exclusively gone online. This greatly reduced their cost, bringing an ease of posting that has significantly increased their numbers. Response time is next to nothing when compared to the good old days of snail mail and post office boxes. Nevertheless, the reality remains that there is still a great deal of frustration associated with ads.

On several occasions, I have asked others about their experiences with ads. Two answers are clear:

First, they work. Placing an ad remains one way to successfully meet interested parties. There is no doubt about that. I met Patrick through an ad, as well as many other men, who remain good friends to this day.

The other response is that using ads is genuinely exasperating. The number of dead end alleys one must traverse, before finding one or two productive responses, can be quite daunting. This experience seems universal.

Ads can get many responses, with few actual actions. A great many of your responses to people answering your ad will go completely unanswered. Many others, who will return your reply, will only do so once or twice. A great number of responders will quickly prove they are merely looking and not looking for you.

Still, play the numbers game you must, though I will again remind you that looking nearer to home in places (bars, munches, clubs) where real people meet face to face is still the best way to make fruitful contact.

Ads ought to be a combination of words and photos. The text part needs to include your stats, what you are seeking, what you have to offer, and a way to respond to your ad. Pictures, though optional, greatly increase the likelihood of an answer, especially face shots, though it is understandable that many people don't want to run the risk of putting their photo in as public a space as the Internet.

Before placing an ad, a bit of preparation will go a long way toward making the process easier. First off, rent either a post office box or get an e-mail address (such as from Yahoo or AOL) that you will use for replies to your ads. Doing so allows you to preserve some kind of privacy and anonymity — not a bad idea in these days of identity theft. You will also have to get a few current pictures of yourself and have them converted to j-pegs for posting with your ad.

Pictures need not be sexually revealing, though if they are, that does help — if you have the kind of body that bears revealing. They need not be of professional quality; if you only have paper copies you can have them scanned by a friend or at a local service, such as Kinko's. If you are too embarrassed to ask a friend or a clerk to help you with this, then you would be well advised to ask yourself if you are ready to conduct your search. The facts prove that including a picture, when possible, greatly increases your response rate. Many readers will not answer an online ad that doesn't include a photo.

Without digressing into a tirade, it's a simple fact that if you must remain deeply closeted in this venture to find a partner, then you probably ought not be looking for a partner. I am not opposed to protecting privacy or using discretion, but advertising works. Without advertising your desire for a master or a slave, you're not going to get much further than solo play. Wishing will not make your prospect ring your doorbell, collar in hand.

In those good old days, publishers charged to run your ad by the word or the number of letters/lines in the ad, giving rise to the use of a great number of abbreviations. Though there still are some space limitations, most of them are quite generous and have ceased to be a serious consideration. Still, you are liable to see (and use) some popular abbreviations, such as FF, CBT, D/s, BDSM, flagging red (or some other color), etc. Again, if these don't mean anything to you, it's time you put down this book and meet us in real time, learn about our vocabulary and mores, and come back when you know what it is that we do (WIITWD).

Your text, to begin, needs to be accurate. Fudging your weight, age, health, and/or availability only means that the reader you have deceived is going to be pissed when the truth is known, and it will be known. Even using euphemisms doesn't quite cut it. "Mature" can mean one thing to a twenty year old, another to a sixty year old. Stats, then, should include your actual age, weight, height, waist, and other physical and personality characteristics that describe you accurately.

If you have gotten this far, I hope you have an idea of what it is that you want in the partner you are seeking, as in the next part of the ad you have to write it down succinctly. Is it a master, a daddy, a mistress, a slave, a boy, or a dog? Is it a combination? Are you open to several alternatives? And what kind of person are you seeking? What stats should they have?

It is painfully obvious here that you need to be careful in what you seek. The more limits you place in writing, the more people you will discourage from answering you. For that reason, more flexibility will bring more productivity; therefore, a wider range of specifications is encouraged. This, though, must be balanced by the reality of what you are truly seeking. If you must have a 24 year old master, then say so, with the understanding that a perfectly fine 25 year old Dom will most likely not answer your ad.

Other considerations that ought to be included are your availability to travel, to relocate, and to meet the terms of the other, such as versatility, part-time play, and sexual activity. If you have definite limits, include them now, such as D/D free (must be disease and drug free) or no cigarettes, alcohol, or penetration. If there are some serious considerations that may be a negative (such as your HIV status), you might keep that out of the ad, but be quick to let your responders know early on in your mutual fact-finding. On the other hand, putting it in the ad will get your point made more quickly and avoid any appearance of deception.

Your need to take care that your ad be factually correct and not give the false impression that you neither have more (or less) experience than is factual, nor that you are willing to do things that, in fact, you won't do.

A helpful way to write your ad is to collect ads of others that seem to reflect what you are seeking and ads of those whom you find attractive. Analyze them for keywords and examples of how you might write your ad. Text that complements — for instance, the ads of masters that you find attractive (i.e., he uses the word "domestic") — ought to echo the same characteristics. Write some ads for yourself and let them rest for a day or two. Then, go back and review them before you post them, as a day later you may see that what your first wrote may need revision.

When you arrive at what you think is your best attempt, let several scene-friendly friends critique it for you. You will be amazed at what others see and don't see in the ad that you think is perfect.

Once the ad is placed, gauge how well it works for you. If your responses are dismal, go back to the drawing board and ascertain how you might change it to improve your response rate. Initial responses to your ad can be conducted via e-mail, but I strongly encourage that you quickly move to phone calls in order to expedite the exchange of information, as well as weed out the cyber-cruisers, who will only waste your time.

The Interview

To begin this section with the words "The Interview" is somewhat misleading because interviewing your applicant is seldom a one-time, cut and dry process. Actually, the interview process begins when you ask the first question, and ends when you have come to some resolution — either of enslavement, friendship, or a parting of the ways. In any case, interviewing is the simple practice of fact-finding and as such, is an integral part of negotiating the relationship.

I include interviewing in this chapter, rather than the next, however, since we often begin interviewing before we begin the more serious process of finding agreement on the details of the scene or life that we are seeking to create. Still, I cannot emphasize too strongly enough that interviewing — fact-finding — is the beginning of the process of negotiation.

As I've written earlier, interviewing is a two-way encounter, even if it seems that one partner, the master applicant, has a greater say in the process than the other. Once again, let me affirm that I believe the two involved in the interview should interview as equals, since both must have enough information to make an informed decision. Whether, in fact, the interview is as equals or as a master-to-be and slave-to-be, it remains important that the dialogue allow each the freedom of full expression and understanding. If either applicant feels inhibited in the discussion, it will be less fruitful and effective.

This isn't always understood in the reality of the process. Too often, applicants (both master and slave) fail to ask the right questions or very many questions at all. They, therefore, seldom gain a complete picture of the person they are considering for a long-term relationship.

Ideally, both partners have a set of questions, based upon their desire and understanding of mastery and slavery, that will guide

60

their questioning. Just as an interview for a job is usually based on a written job description, published requirements, such as education and experience, and the nuances of the needs determined by the employer and employee, so too should an interview leading to enslavement have similar resources at its beginning. That has been the purpose of this book thus far: to give you some ideas as to what you will want to know before you meet.

In reality, the interview will most likely be a series of conversations conducted in various ways over a period of time. Let me cite a recent example: I met Tom at a Chicago Hellfire Club Party. I found him attractive and articulate, and noted that he was looking for a master. With that information in mind, I handed him my personal card, which contained my name, phone number, and e-mail address, and told him I would like to talk to him about his search.

He then responded two days later with an e-mail. After two or three e-mails were exchanged, which, in fact, confirmed we were both interested, I invited him to call me. Thus began the interview process. Some six or eight phone calls later, we had plans for the interview to become more personal. That meant he would visit me in my home for a weekend to experience slavery under my mastery.

During these interviews, I have asked about his professional life, his family, his coming out, his interest in slavery, his experiences as a gay man and as a submissive. We have talked about his feelings, his social life, and his desires. For my part, I have talked about my experiences, my ideas concerning mastery and slavery, my household situation, and my fantasy to own multiple slaves.

Areas appropriate for the interviewers to consider include finances, health, fantasy, career, family relationships, education, experience in BDSM, availability, personality, hobbies, time spent with other masters, sexual and fetish preferences, limits, and spiritual beliefs. In actuality, no topic is off-limits in the long-run, if we are talking about creating a long-term relationship.

On the other hand, the depth of the questioning and the answers given are determined by the stage at which the couple-to-be find themselves in the process of negotiation. For that reason, for example, I may ask early on if the candidate is generally free of burdensome debt or can afford to travel to meet me. It would not be appropriate to ask for his Social Security Number or his credit card accounts, though I might need to know those things sometime before he moves in with me.

In conducting interviews, I am careful to encourage my applicants to ask me the same questions I ask them. If I need to know the status of their health, for instance, they probably ought to know mine as well. This is all part of developing rapport and gaining enough information to know that my prospect can be trusted and is a candidate with the qualities that I am seeking. In fact, the more he knows about me, the higher the possibility (one hopes) that he will trust me. Trust is the basis for our relationship and we must take care to lay a good basis for trust to exist and grow; hence, the need for good interviewing techniques.

At an educational seminar several years ago, I was given a list of dos and don'ts concerning active listening. I am sorry not to have a reference for this list:

- Do make encouraging remarks (I see, uh huh, right...)
- Do give nonverbal acknowledgement (nod, match facial expressions, open and relaxed body posture, eye contact).
- Do invite more information if required for understanding.
- Do reflect what you observe or hear and how you believe the speaker feels.
- Don't interrupt.
- Don't change the subject.
- Don't rehearse in your head.
- Don't interrogate.
- Don't teach or lecture.

The success of your interview will determine the timing of the next step: meeting face to face. There is the need here for a balance. Arrange to meet when you feel you have learned enough about one another to get more seriously involved in the process. Too soon may lead to a meeting that goes nowhere. Delay it for too long a time and you most likely will never get past talking.

The First Meeting

The quality and type of first meeting that you and your applicant will have greatly depends upon several factors, such as geography, level of trust, and sexual limits. It is common, therefore, for applicants who have yet to meet, but live in geographical proximity to one another, to simply get together in a neutral location for coffee or a drink, while they ask relatively easy questions. Such meetings can have little or no agenda and often hold no expectations for more than meeting. On the other hand, if the applicants already know one another, the first meeting may be more intense, more personal, and of longer duration.

Likewise, if applicants are geographically separated by distance, the first meeting may not take place until there has been a great deal of dialogue, preferably by phone. Once the meeting is agreed upon, a location is picked, and arrangements are made. I will often invite the slave-applicant to my home for a weekend, with the understanding that if our time together indicates that we won't be pursuing a relationship, then he is welcome to stay in my home as a tourist, though some might prefer to simply go home sooner.

One of my practices here has a lot to do with expectations. Since one never knows how the first encounter will progress, I make sure expectations are reasonable and flexible. On more than one occasion, my applicant has realized within the first few minutes that we weren't going to get very far with this meeting. Better have a Plan B or you're going to be in big trouble.

Clicking

The primary value of the first meeting, over and beyond the information gathered by conversing, is that both parties will begin to have a much better sense as to whether or not they will "click." As I review the list of men and women who have become significant others in my life, each of them shares a very important experience with me. Simply put, we clicked. I liked Ann (whom I married) the evening I met her. I fell in love with Bart immediately. In my heart, I became Master Lynn's slave about 90 seconds after meeting him. I knew Patrick would be my slave the first night we met.

I could say that about lots of friends and fuck-buddies as well. Though clicking is certainly not the only criteria upon which to base a relationship, it is an important one. Unfortunately, it is a criterion to which we in the Leather world don't seem to pay very much attention — as if the right chemistry isn't very important when it comes to kink. I have chosen a word as obscure as clicking to differentiate it from the word love, since it's not always a case of "falling in love," though that may certainly be a significant part of the experience.

A recent e-mail gives you an idea about what I mean. A man who is exploring his submissive side wrote: He took "me to a place that I hadn't been before. With him, he led me and I touched that emotional / spiritual place that I had been seeking.... That experience is one of those life events I will treasure, as do most with a spiritual happening. Prior to playing with him, and doing 'slap and tickle' SM, I had not even had an experience of medium intensity. He didn't know that. There were no limits discussed because for whatever reason I knew I didn't need them with him....I believe the trust between us was the catapult for the experience."

Here we have a novice to SM, meeting a very experienced player, trusting him immediately, and playing roughly for several hours with no prior negotiations, no safe words, and (later) no regrets. How can this be? They clicked.

Now, there are lots of reasons "to click" and there is no need to list

63

them as they vary widely among people. What can be said, though, is that it is a mutual experience, basically intuitive, and often fragile. This rapport, elusive and difficult to describe, is what I find missing in so many of our presentations, our writing, and our instructions, formal or not, about Leather.

Now, there is a lot to be said for gaining experience for the sake of experience. You don't have to be in love to let someone drip hot wax on you if you merely want to have that experience. Sex for the sake of sex, mutual masturbation (if you will), needs no emotional or romantic component. Quickies are just that. There are times, too, when the click is one-sided, as when my friend David brought Steven to a party at my place. Steven fell in love with me; I hardly noticed him. It would be nearly a year before we got together, at which time, belatedly, we clicked. Even then, it was more than a year later before I realized I loved him.

This emotional-intuitive response is one way to begin a relationship, but a healthy relationship needs to include other components as well. There needs be a willful and mutual commitment to continue and foster the relationship, and to allow it to also have intellectual, physical, and spiritual dimensions. Infatuation will eventually wear away and there must be a structure in place to sustain the relationship for longer than "the bloom is on the rose."

But before all that happens, we should be mindful of the importance of this kind of rapport, however elusive it might be. What I am struggling to say is that there is a lot more to SM than its technical aspects. Since we can render the technical with words, they take on an importance that overshadows its less concrete aspects. We get all caught up in negotiations, in contracts, in proper techniques and protocols. We begin to act as if they are what is integral and important, as if attending a few workshops makes us a slave or having a certificate makes us a master.

That is not to disparage the fine efforts of those who teach, write, demonstrate, and inform. It is only to put the dogma they espouse into proper perspective. The emotional, romantic, and affectionate aspects of SM may, in fact, be more important than good technique and correct protocol, since without those qualities, our play becomes rote, sterile, and possibly without meaning.

It seems to me that ignoring the emotional component is what leads us down so many "dead end" roads in our search for partners. Have we reached a point where our kinky activity is more important than our partner? Where our physical and sexual needs take priority over our social, emotional, and spiritual ones? It is no wonder that so many searches end in naught. We are investing huge amounts of time and effort into intellectual and/or cyber events, while possibly ignoring how we feel about one another. We build fantasies on a laundry list of qualities that Mr. or Ms. Right will have, without ever answering the questions: "Do you love me?" or "Do I like you?"

Good SM is based upon underlying relationships of trust and commitment, if only for the night. Long-term SM is based on deeper trust and deeper commitment. Though I can't advocate that a relationship be based only on "hitting it off," likewise, you can't build one without doing so. Infatuation is not the end-all; love isn't always enough to make a relationship work. Emotions alone cannot sustain a long-term relationship. Lack of emotions, love-less-ness, and not hitting it off, on the other hand, will ensure that there will be no relationship. What we miss in the chat rooms, in the classifieds, and in the cruising in the bars, is the recognition of the importance of this emotional component — though I hasten to add that at least in the bar scene, there's a chance you'll click.

For that reason, I have begun to shorten the length of time I will devote to cyber-cruising and phone conversations. I am increasingly aware of the need to look my potential partner in the eye, shake his hand, share dinner, and see how he kisses before I get all involved in the practicalities of our next scene.

You see, it's very often the case that the emotional component will, for better or for worse, and much to our surprise, completely overrule any other criteria. I suppose it's the "least expect it" syndrome. All four of my long-term relationships began when I least expected them to, yet each of them held the possibility of becoming very successful relationships. It may not have been according to plan, but it worked.

In any case, the first meeting may include some SM play, initial training of the slave, or only a pleasant conversation. What does transpire is going be at the lead of the dominant, with the consent of the submissive.

The Experiment

Having written some 65 pages about voluntary servitude, it's now time to remind you that it's about developing a physical relationship. Simply put, don't talk each other to death!

For that reason, I insist that our dialogue not last for more than a month. In fact, after observing years of my (mostly) fruitless talking with wannabes, Patrick began to encourage me to meet with an applicant sooner, not later, as it became obvious that there was a general tendency to do nothing more than talk. If talk was all I wanted, I would have joined Toastmasters.

My new policy is to converse until I think that we know each other well enough to meet and then issue an invitation. If the applicant can't visit me, then I politely put him on hold, reminding him that I can be patient and that our dialogue will lessen in intensity until he is ready to commit to meeting me. In some situations, I invite them to meet me at a Leather conference or I volunteer to travel to their homes.

This meeting does hold expectations that it will contain some kind of physical intimacy. Even if you are not looking for a sexual relationship, it is a good idea to spend some time early in the process to experience each other as physical beings. How does your applicant feel dressed in her sissy maid uniform? How does she respond to your whips and crops? What is it like to kiss your master's feet?

These questions are only posed as guidelines. The actual questions, which reflect real experience, will depend upon your (and this word is plural) mutually agreed upon definition of how your future relationship will be structured. There is a reason why this is called "The Experiment," as the purpose of this meeting is to see if you will be able to move beyond talk to action.

I can't speak for you, but for my part I learn a great deal about a prospect when I can look into his eyes, feel how he kisses, and watch how his reaction to the caress of my hand or the touch of my paddle. Give me half an hour in bed with an applicant and I will know quite well if this encounter is the first of many or the simply the end of long dialogue.

I am not saying that this physical encounter has to be a make or break, all or nothing, event. It does provide, however, a great deal of information upon which to evaluate yourselves as fit for one another.

The physical aspects are not only sexual. Are you comfortable in each other's presence? Is her home able to accommodate you? Does her schedule leave time for quality time with each other? Does the life you are witnessing firsthand affirm the promises and descriptions given over the phone or via e-mail?

Evaluation

The way in which I have described this process of finding a partner runs the very real risk that you will conclude that there are actual steps in this process. I have chosen this methodology for organizational reasons, but in reality, the steps are more like phases. The phases, like the myriad of waves in the light spectrum, need be neither discreet nor monochromatic.

Your interviewing will continue even after you've met. You will be evaluating one another throughout the process of getting to know one another, as well as during the negotiating and training phases. Evaluation never ceases, even if it takes on a less critical mode once you have both made some decisions about your future.

I believe that the ongoing evaluation of an applicant is one of the most important phases in becoming a master or a slave. Regrettably, we tend to evaluate poorly, either by continuing down dead-end roads because we desperately want to be enslaved, or by dismissing very good candidates because of issues within ourselves that are not yet resolved.

The first fault, continuing when we ought not, leads to wasted resources at best and, at worse, a miserable relationship that will end. It is understandable that becoming a slave (or a master, for that matter) is a strong, heartfelt desire. Many of those who have such an ambition will understandably do almost anything to achieve it. For that reason, it is important to remember that having no relationship is very much preferable to being in a bad one.

Continuing evaluation means that we look before we leap and that when we leap, we keep our eyes wide open. It means that we have to be honest with ourselves and our applicant, not glossing over red or yellow flags, but plainly recognizing them for what they are. As my applicant and I become more serious and approach certain milestones, such as a first visit or the signing of a short-term contract, I often pause to share my hesitations with them. I am frank and honest about how my evaluation of our potential is progressing and I encourage them to do the same.

Note that what is evaluated is our progress. I am not judging the other as an individual. Instead, I am weighing the possibility, probability, and reliability of our having a mutually created relationship. Remember, here, the second part of slavery's definition. Just because we may not be suited for one another does not mean that both of us aren't well suited for a master/slave relationship with someone else.

Just as I am honest in my evaluation of us, I need to be the same in my evaluation of myself. Are the negatives that I am seeing simply a result of my own projections, fears, or unreasonable expectations? One applicant, for instance, was quick to dismiss me as a potential candidate because I lived in a city where it snowed. It took a year of frustrating searching on his part to conclude that perhaps he would have to leave the land of sun and hurricanes in order to live his life as a slave. A year later, I was back on his short list.

I write this because a surprising number of searchers are unable to see that their definitions, their expectations, or their criteria are incredibly unrealistic. Personal ads are filled with fruitless requests seeking that under 25, athletic, educated, sexy, completely submissive, no-limit slave, who will solve every problem a master might have. On the slave's part, the search for the master who will serve him breakfast in the cage every morning, provide for every need while the slave is kept hidden from the cares of the world in the dungeon, or take him away from every responsibility he ever had, is just as frivolous a search.

Evaluation is one of those two-way streets, to be sure. Like the equality of each in interviewing, so too it is the responsibility of each to evaluate.

I suggest that an effective way to evaluate is to spend time making a list of the pros and cons your prospect and you bring to the bargaining table. On one side of the page, list all the reasons the other person is the right choice for you. On the other, list the negatives that you see or suspect. Which side of the page has the longer list? Which list holds the more important reasons? Prioritize each list as well, as perhaps a real strong "pro" will easily outweigh several less important negatives, or there may be some negatives that are deal breakers.

You'll have to decide on the merits of each characteristic, including its importance and its weight. I can neither list all the pros that will be meaningful, nor all the cons that are important, but some examples may be helpful.

On the plus side, consider: stability, consistency, references, attractiveness, experience, physical, emotional, and cultural compatibility. Do the same with the negatives, as well. Use them as discussion points.

Let your applicant know what is causing your hesitation. Good dialogue about these things could, in fact, quickly and easily eliminate the red flag completely. You see, sometimes the red flags appear because we have misunderstood one another. Our ability to evaluate isn't always as well honed as we might hope, either. For those reasons, give each other a chance to explain. "Hard" negatives might include addictions, incapacitating health issues, family obligations, impatience, haughtiness, stinginess, and inflexibility.

Be careful, too, how you share these negatives. Remain positive in your speech and demeanor. Begin the conversation by listing the pluses so that your applicant will know that you are not attacking him or her, only seeking to improve both your chances for success. Likewise, don't take their hesitations personally, as they have as much right to their feelings as you do to yours.

There are two characteristics that one might also use as a strong basis for evaluation. The first of these relies on the sure axiom that "Actions speak louder than words."

Does your master-to-be do what he says he will regarding replying in a timely manner, calling you at the hour he has appointed, or doing something which he has said he would do? Likewise, have you as a submissive-to-be obeyed the things you were told to do? Quite frankly, many masters give small tasks to determine the slave-applicant's ability to follow orders. I have asked applicants to send me pictures or resumes, to call at a specific and agreed upon time, to send me a postcard, read a web page, or write in a journal. Failure to comply speaks volumes. As a therapist who counseled me once said, "When a client says one thing and does another, I always listen to what they do." What, in fact, are your actions saying? What does your lack of obedience prove? As I wrote in chapter two, "The M/s relationship can be best evaluated by the extent to which control is expressed in action." The same can be said for the slave-applicant. He or she can be best evaluated by the response to the master's control, as expressed in obedience.

Another, and similar, characteristic that speaks loudly is to note your applicant's priorities. If his life is too busy to make time for you during the finding, negotiating, and evaluating phases, it will be too busy for you when you attempt to live in a 24/7 relationship. If a proposed meeting date can only be scheduled for some time considerably later; if meetings, phone calls, or other events are often postponed or cancelled; if the applicant often arrives late, having been delayed by something else; you have an applicant who is not seriously looking to own or be owned. That person is probably only wasting your time and hers.

My response to just such an applicant is to advise him or her to contact me when able to make the process of enthrallment a higher priority. Needless to say, I have had to learn to be very patient.

None of the above is meant to imply that I don't cut my applicants some slack, or that you shouldn't do the same. The world in which we live is a busy place and rearranging one's life is never an easy matter.

References

Though we tend to use them a great deal less than in past decades, it still behooves applicants to ask for and check references. This is a rule mostly ignored, but using it — especially before any commitments are made — could spare both parties a lot of grief.

If nothing else, the lack of references indicates either a loner status or the lack of real time experience with our community. For me, either of those is a serious red flag.

Don't hesitate to ask for references before you begin to make a commitment. References are certainly helpful when it comes to ascertaining the suitability of an applicant who is at a distance or for one where you suspect, but cannot confirm, a "fatal flaw." For example, I would have saved myself considerable grief if I had asked for references on a candidate who did eventually move in. In the interview process, I was rushed because he kept telling me about his dysfunctional roommate, who wanted him out of the house. A simple conversation with the roommate might well have told me that I didn't want him to move in with me either.

On the other hand, references are much simpler than we think. It's not as if the reference has to know the applicant's whole life history. Good references include anyone who has met the applicant and can vouch that they are a real person involved in the scene. An event producer can confirm, for example, that he or she attended a seminar, a fuck-buddy can attest to their experience, even a landlord can tell you that the person live where he says he lives.

All of this can be done without letting on that the reason you want to know about them has to do with SM. Even a discreet phone call to them at work proves that they are employed.

One of the purposes of references is to help you avoid the "loner." Time and again, investigation into problems with BDSM can be traced to the fact that the perpetrator was a loner, often completely unknown to the other players in his or her region, not a member of a real-time club, munch, or organization and certainly not subscribing to any of our codes or mores, and especially prone to avoiding both "safe, sane, and consensual" and "trust, honor, and respect."

Place your bets on the known entities. Leave the loners to find a community and lose their loner status before you meet them, not after.

Upping the Ante

My grandmother, Rose, was an avid poker player. I can't remember a Thanksgiving, Christmas, or Easter dinner that didn't end in a card game, or a picnic that didn't include "penny ante." In fact, as a child my grandmother had a hard and fast rule that she would never babysit for my brother and me on Saturday nights. As important as her grandchildren were, they played second fiddle to that regular card game. It should be no surprise, then, that part of my process involves "upping the ante."

We are seeking, I hope, a long-term relationship of dominance and submission. On the other hand, I fully recognize that we are equals in the process of interviewing and negotiating. How, then, do we move from peers to master and slave? The answer is that over time we "up the ante."

The first upping, then, is when I tell the candidate to call me "Sir." Jack is fine when we begin, but there comes a time, based on the slave-applicant's willingness, that I will ask him to call me Sir. Later in the process, I may ask that he be naked when we talk on the phone or that he kneel. In any case, it is a slow process of enthrallment that does two things. Notice that my upping depends upon the candidate's willingness. As we converse, each of us gets a sense of how well the fledgling relationship is growing and how fast we can grow it. There are two reasons for our becoming slowly, but increasingly, dominant and submissive.

First, it gives the candidate a "taste" of what it is like to be submissive to me. That taste is meant to help both of us evaluate our possibilities. After all, if a person can't remember to say Sir, then we're going to have problems.

That is the second reason. Upping the ante gives me something to evaluate. This can be a two-way street, as well. If your prospective dominant is too casual for you or (heaven forbid) too strict, upping the ante (or not) may well tell you something.

Patrick Reflects: How to Find a Master

Personally I think that the most important part of finding a master is done before you begin actively looking. Here's my formula for success, though it comes with no guarantees or promises.

The First Rule: Time

From the point when you figure out that the idea of slavery turns you on, to the point when you enter a 24/7 relationship, there needs to be some significant time and thought and energy expended. And "time" is the important part of the equation. Don't think you can "discover" slavery and immediately move in with a Master. It may sexually arouse you, but it doesn't mean it's right for you. It takes time to really understand what slavery involves, how it can enhance your life, and how well suited you are to it. Only time is going to help you determine this. Time is a good test to see if the desire is there when the "hard" or "wet" goes away.

So what do you do with this time? First of all, begin with yourself.

What this means is that most of the resources you'll need in this search are found within yourself, not on the Internet. Figuring out who you are, AND what you want, AND what you are ready for, are much more difficult tasks than you think. In fact, you will probably think your search is complete, when in reality, it's just beginning. Any time sex is involved, we tend to rush things.

Think things through before you go off half-cocked, or fully-cocked, for that matter (which is the only time many people contemplate being a slave). To do otherwise will increase the negative experiences you'll have. It can also give you a bad reputation and create bad habits. In this day and age of free and easily changed e-mail addresses, it's easy to hide behind screen names that encourage dishonesty, and a lack of consideration and basic politeness. Aliases can be cancelled on a whim and thus, encourage further disingenuous behavior.

You can end your first attempt on a whim or you can think before you lead someone on. We are talking about finding yourself a master, someone you want to let have some measure of control over your life; so, you'd better do some careful thinking about this. It involves some complicated decisions; it's about being a part of another person's life.

What do you have to offer?

Not material belongings. I mean the less tangible ones that describe you body, mind and soul. It's not just that you offer to serve and be obedient, because anyone can offer those two qualities. Ask any master or top how often they've heard those undelivered promises and you'll understand why this is not enough.

You have to be willing to offer more: proper attitude, pliable nature, clear thinking, a reasonably healthy body, a life not in complete shambles.... The list can go on and on. You might not have all of those qualities, but those you do have should be offered. And, if the list is not very long, you should wait to offer yourself until it is. After all, if you REALLY want to be a slave, the wait will be worth it.

Seriously look at yourself...

...in the mirror, on an emotional level, on a career and social level, sexually, and on any other level you can think of. What improvements can be made? How can you take what is there and make it better?

You don't have to be buff and beautiful, and if you spend too much time and thought on that part of yourself, you'll fool yourself into thinking that's all that matters. I'd like to think that any master would be happy to have proper attitude over knockout looks, but unfortunately, that's not the way it always works. It's going to be up to you to make sure there is more to you than appearance and that you find a master who is smart enough to look more intently than skin deep.

Age is not a disqualifying factor either, though it might affect what you are capable of, and who your master ends up being. Years may make it more difficult, but not impossible. There's nothing you can do about the time you've wasted getting to this point; so, work with what time you've left for yourself and make the most of it, understanding that waiting until parents have died or retirement comes creates limits, but not necessarily roadblocks.

Likewise, it is unreasonable to think that things such as getting in shape, losing weight or kicking drugs are things you want your future master to make you do. Your master can only make you do what you are capable of doing yourself. Surrender to your servitude as the best you can be and you will be seen as serious, determined and worthy.

Surrender yourself as less than you can be and you immediately start off in the wrong direction. Your future master deserves nothing less than the best you can give, and once this is offered, your master can take it and improve upon it, making you the slave he (or she) desires you to be.

What traumas are you experiencing in your life? It's seldom a good idea to make a major decision for your life when it is in turmoil. You don't rush out and become a slave because life has dealt you an unexpected or heavy blow. It isn't a matter of thinking you have no other choice. Turmoil blinds you to many things and can make bad situations seem pretty good. If you become a slave because you think you have no other choice, then you will quit being a slave as soon as you think of another alternative.

Being a slave doesn't mean you are merely adding some sexy fun to the many other things in your life. It will most certainly mean reordering those other things, giving them a less important place to make room for something... someone... more important.

Look at these soul searching questions:

What kind of attitude do you have? Attitude, after all, is of primary importance. It's a mistake to assume your master will force you to submit. No master has the energy it takes to do that all of the time, and there will be plenty of "special" things they will want you to submit to that will take enough of their energy. Abduction, prisoner/warden, coercion, forced servitude: these are interesting fantasies, but not valid realities, at least when we are talking about voluntary servitude.

Is the list of things you disapprove of, or have difficulty accepting, longer than the list of things that you approve of or like? This will be a sign of problems and may be an indicator that perhaps slavery is not a life you'll enjoy. I've always liked the way Shakespeare put it: "Being your slave, what should I do but tend upon the hours and times of your desire?"§ It's rule #1 around our house and is both a serious expectation on Sir's part and a devoted commitment on my part. It isn't about selfishness or my mere obedience; it's about devotion to the ideals that shape our relationship and commitment. As this indicates, as a slave your thoughts should be more on what it is your master or mistress desires than what you want, and the more things you don't like, the harder it will be to give that kind of devotion.

In the same vein, is the list of things you want done to you longer than the list of things you will do for your master? A slave isn't a dome queen; being a slave isn't about "make me feel good." It's about finding contentment in being there for the pleasure of your master or mistress.

How do you approach decision making for yourself? Are you more dependent than submissive, or more obsessive than committed? How

§ Shakespeare, William, *Sonnet LVII*

do you handle responsibility? Why should your future master take on someone who can't manage an unmanageable life? Moving your problems in on your master shows a lack of respect for yourself, and a greater lack of respect for your future master. Think about it for a moment. Would you want to have to solve your master's problems or have to straighten out his life? That isn't to say that there are some things you just can't make happen on your own, and you recognize that a strong hand will help you resolve them. How few and how big those problems are will all play a part in your success with your future master.

What is it that you want out of life? Is it compatible with being a slave? What is your relationship with your family like and how much will you be able to tell them about someone new in your life? What responsibilities to others do you have and will you be able to deal with them appropriately if you become a slave? What about your job or career? How will you manage that while a slave?

These are all valid questions that you need to ask yourself. If you don't know all of the answers, you need to at least have started yourself on the road to finding them.

There is a lot of misunderstanding about what a slave is. The inexperienced and uninitiated grab onto every erotic fantasy that tickles their loins and think that is what constitutes slavery. The fantasy of being caged all of the time is quite attractive to some; for them, nothing would be more liberating than to find a sadistic, dominant top to stick them in a cage, feed them dog-food, and do rude things with their orifices. But they have no clue what it would really be like, and that's not slavery. Slavery means serving, rather than being served. Most thrive on the fantasy of slavery, but fail with its reality. Becoming a slave can be freeing, liberating and satisfying, but it is also about obedience, service and devotion, even when your loins are no longer feeling tickled.

Overcome your fears.

Fear is what stops people from moving from fantasy to reality. What would friends say? What would family say? What if you were laughed at? Even fear of what would happen if someone made the fantasy a reality. Fear is a powerful thing, and the sooner you conquer it, the more satisfying your search will be. Conquering it allows you to devote your time and energy towards the search, rather than the fear. That is why time is going to be necessary and why I can say that it will be time well spent.

Rule Two: Explore and Gain Experience
I've seen it over and over again. Individuals fantasize what slavery will be like. They dream about it. They surf the web looking for every

reference they can find. They even use the anonymity of the web to try to explore what it would be like without making any kind of commitment. But they are afraid or unwilling to actually experience it.

At some point, they reach a decision. They are going to take that step and become a slave and move in right away. The problem is that they have no real clue about what it is they want. They haven't taken the time to gain experience, to know what the difference is between being a bottom and being a slave. They don't know what happens beyond the bondage and fucking (or before it for that matter). It's amazing to me how many e-mails Sir gets from people who have no experience in bondage, corporal punishment, or even what kinky sex is like. Yet they want to go from 0 to 100 immediately, as though there is nothing in-between.

If you've never been flogged, shouldn't you experience it in a less committed way than by giving yourself totally to someone and then finding out what it's about, and that you don't like it? Or what happens if your master ties you down, decides to fist fuck you and you freak out because you don't even know what fist fucking is?

You don't decide you want to play the violin and start out by applying to the Chicago Symphony. It takes lessons, and practice, and recitals, and contests, and auditions... a lot of work and experience before you are ready for that big step. It wouldn't look good if all you could do is play a string version of chopsticks.

Exploring allows you to understand what the lifestyle is all about. It allows you to find out what bondage is like, how it feels to be confined in a sleep sack for hours on end, the difference between being flogged and being single-tailed. You have a chance to learn what it is that you like and what you don't like, what makes you hard and what you find a bore. It helps confirm the depths of your interest in the lifestyle. Once you've gained experience in what kinky people do, you will have learned HOW they do it and get a glimpse of what it will be like to be someone's slave. You'll give yourself to a master or mistress for a brief time and see what it feels like to lose control and independence for that brief period. If that experience makes you hot, you can take a step further, for a longer period of time, to see if it still fits.

Exploring gives you an inkling of what commitment you are capable. Then, and only then, are you ready to begin finding a master — that special person to whom you want to commit, who you want to mold you and make you into the kind of slave he or she finds useful.

After Reading Activities
Answer the following in your journal:

What special characteristics do you think your master ought to have? How is he different from the masters you have met thus far? What special characteristics do you have that make you unique?

Think about your friends and lovers (past and present) and list the things about them that you found attractive. Why?

What hard limits do you have concerning your living as a slave? What characteristics must your master have? Are they reasonable and attainable?

Make a list of questions that you might ask your prospective master. For ideas, you may want to search the Internet for some sample questionnaires or use the one in Appendix B. Rate the importance of each question on a scale of one to ten.

Write an ad searching for your partner. Show it to three scene-friendly people and ask them to evaluate it. Based on their ideas, re-write it, making sure it still suits you.

If you haven't done it yet, gather a list of references that you can give a prospective partner. Check with the references to be sure that it's OK to use their names. Only include phone numbers or e-mail addresses (you're going to have include one or the other) with their permission.

4

Negotiating the Relationship

It takes two to tango.[*]

Though we seldom think of testing when it comes to BDSM, it is, in fact, an important part of what we do. We prefer to use the term negotiation, but in reality, Leather folk spend a lot of time testing each other to determine the propriety of entering into a relationship.

That last sentence is loaded with caveats. First off, relationship isn't capitalized. We test for the purpose of having a one-time scene, just as much as we test for the purpose of becoming long-term partners. Clubs test pledges before they admit them as members; masochists test sadists before they allow themselves to be tied to a St. Andrew's cross. Pro-Dommes test clients before they accept payment for a session. If you are doubtful of these things, simply reread this paragraph while substituting the word negotiate for the word test.

As with most tests, they are a two-way street. I know that my students seldom think that their teacher is being tested, but I am. My coordinator keeps an eye out to ensure that I meet the requirements in the syllabus, and my chairperson reads student evaluations of my performance each semester. I was "tested" by the administration before I was hired to ensure that I knew my pedagogy and my content area.

Likewise, and this is seldom noted, bottoms test prospective tops. They need to, in order to ensure both their safety and their pleasure.

For that reason, I am adamant that all negotiations need to be open, honest, and without the constriction of roles. If the master-to-be thinks he or she is superior in the negotiations, then it is going to be less effective. If the bottom thinks he has no right to ask questions to determine the top's suitability, he is grossly in error. If we do not operate with full disclosure,

---

[*] This American idiom was taught to me by my mother.

77

on both sides, if we do not respect one another enough to be honest in our answers and forthright in our questions, then the relationship — for however long we hope it to last — is crippled from the start.

For a slave-applicant, for instance, not to have any questions of his master-applicant, is at best a shaky approach, and at its worst, dangerous territory. The primary reason why so many relationships fail, or scenes are less than satisfactory, is that we don't gather enough information before we plunge head-long into them. That may be one of the reasons that arranged marriages seemed to work: the parents at least knew what questions to ask.

The questions are determined by our expectations. I don't need to know as much about a person with whom I am going to play in a public dungeon or club house, as I do about someone who I am going to ask to move in with me. Still, there are questions that must be asked in each scenario.

For that reason, we Leather men developed (and used to use) long questionnaires that covered as many bases as we felt we needed. Mine[†] included topics of health, geography, expectations, and experience. I asked about references, family, employment, education, hobbies, finances, past relationships, and, of course, fetishes. I sought (and still do) to know about the applicant's desire and experience in fucking, sucking, rimming, whipping, bondage, fisting, pain, service, body worship, obedience, readiness, and ability to meet and eventually relocate.

My applicants ought to know the same about me. That's why it remains such a mystery that I get asked so few questions when I am interviewing a candidate, though their lack of questions ought to give me a clue that I shouldn't expect much from the applicant. It is less of a mystery why those few questions revolve around sex; in talking with lots of these applicants, you'd never know that sex is only part of the equation.

Now, if the testing is only for a scene, I can understand there is no need to discuss plans for one's retirement. Still, we ought to ask, "Who's going to pay for what when we meet?" I will never forget a dinner with a slave-applicant that I had some twenty years ago. New as I was to all of this, I had never asked who was going to pay the restaurant bill. After dinner, to my surprise, I learned that the evening's host was me. Luckily, I had cash in my wallet. It was the last time I failed to ask that question before we ordered off the menu.

I have also learned to bring up the hard questions sooner rather than later. I am tired of getting all hot and sweaty over the newest possibility, only to find they are in a monogamous relationship and only looking to chat. I want to know sooner, not later, whether this conversation

† See Appendix B for suggestions for a questionnaire.

has a chance of ending in a pleasant tryst. The only way to ascertain that is to ask the right questions and to listen to how vague or specific their answers are.

Lest you think that the test is only oral, be assured that it's not. One can tell a great deal about where a scene is headed by the first hug and the first kiss. When I go to kiss someone, and the person turns his or her lips away from mine, one hell of a lot of information is communicated silently and effectively. In that regard, testing is a continuing process, until all the details are arranged and the end is achieved.

There are many other opportunities to know a prospect's true potential as well. Is he or she known by others who can be references? Have they attended seminars or demos? Are they employed and where? Are they accomplished in non-sexual areas of their life? What do they think of when they are masturbating? When was the last time they were fucked and by whom? What cultural, sporting, and social events interest them? Do you share likes in music, entertainment, food, etc.?

Experience counts, too, though it is not always a necessary ingredient. Novices can, after all, be fun to teach. That possibility, though, must also be proven. Is your prospective partner teachable? Reasonable? Willing to communicate? Open to change? Is there honesty about limitations and their level of experience?

One of the most important indicators of success is follow-through. When I ask an applicant to call at such and such a time, I expect them to do so. When I ask them to make a list of questions, I want to know that they've got the list handy the next time I call. I look for them to communicate, if they are serious about what our future might hold. If negotiating isn't a priority, then I'm not about to waste my time chasing them.

Let me repeat this for emphasis: One of the most important indicators of success is follow-through. Finding a master is not an easy process; it is counterproductive to waste your time with those whose lack of response only delays the inevitable. Move on to find an applicant — master or slave — who is serious enough about the search, that the possibility of success exists for both of you.

Conversely, every time your applicant's response is positive and timely, you will know you are moving in the right direction. When they are courteous, pleasant, inquisitive, and receptive, I know we are one step closer to a successful encounter. The final exam, after all, is seldom a make or break moment. Instead, the whole process indicates a potential for success. Understand the process as a test and you will help create the atmosphere for success.

The Nature of Negotiations

Trade unions, nations, families, businesses, neighbors, politicians, and everyone else, for that matter, negotiate. What is it? It's the "conferring with one another in order to come to terms or reach an agreement." Agreement, understandably is a good thing, especially when it comes to sex, commitment, and a host of other considerations about living.

Negotiation takes many forms, even to the point that we talk about "negotiating a curve." Closer to our BDSM home, our subculture has long encouraged and taught negotiation as a necessary prelude to having a scene; limits must be ascertained, health and experience levels considered, and general agreement reached on how, when, and where the scene will take place.

As chief negotiator for our teachers' union, I've learned that "interest-based" bargaining[‡] is quite helpful. Whereas traditional bargaining tends to be rather confrontational, interest-based bargaining is much more appropriate for what we do. We are, after all, seeking a win-win situation. By looking for areas of mutual interest while negotiating, we are more liable to make it work for both parties, rather than compromising in such a way that neither of us gets what we really want.

On the other hand, compromise is sometimes necessary and not always a bad thing, though I would caution against compromising those things that really are important to you. In the long run, the compromise could possibly come back to haunt you with regrets and eventually bring to naught all your negotiations.

Negotiation between partners is an ongoing and progressive task. Early negotiations simply establish interest and gather facts. As you progress, you will have to refine your discussions and hone in on specific matters of concern. Unlike negotiating for a scene, negotiations will take place over a period of time and will include many of the same topics found in your questionnaire.

More importantly, they will have to include serious considerations about finances, careers, and living arrangements. These will be about specifics, too. How do you consolidate two households? What do you do about the pets, your family, your retirement funds? What timetable will you agree upon for becoming master and slave? Is this a right now thing, in three months, or next year? The list of questions will be seemingly endless.

Don't be daunted by the task. Remember that you eat an elephant one bite at a time. If you take your negotiations slowly and piecemeal,

‡   For more information on this approach see Fisher, Roger, Ury, William, and Patton, Bruce, *Getting to Yes: Negotiating Agreement Without Giving In*, 2nd Edition, Penguin Books, ISBN 0140157352, 1991.

allowing yourselves plenty of time to get to know one another and learning to enjoy one another, you will arrive at agreement much sooner than you think.

Remember that your negotiations need to find mutual agreement. Don't let yourself be convinced to do something that you would rather not do. It is better to walk away than it is to give in and regret doing so later.

In all of this, remember to have fun.

Petitions

Petitions of one sort or another have been a part of our community for a long time: Pro-Dommes, clubs, contact groups, and cruising men have used them in various ways for years. Simply put, a petition is a means for an applicant to put on paper his or her desire to enter into a relationship with someone. The piece of paper and the ink have no real value or power in themselves, but rendering one's thoughts on paper helps to clarify them for you and make them clearer for your partner.

Not only does the writing help clarify our desires, but the writing of a petition deliberately slows down the process, allowing for mutual evaluation. Additionally, I have found that the exercise of committing things to writing is a powerful help in clarifying our meaning, our desire, and the commitment itself. Written thoughts are also more permanent, so that their intent isn't forgotten. The very act of committing the details to paper gives all concerned a chance to grapple with their meaning, implications, and expectations so all parties have a better understanding of what the prospective relationship entails.

In this context, at a minimum, a good petition contains the request to join — a declaration to participate according to the "rules," and usually, the signatures of the applicant and those sponsoring him or her.

Most social organizations have some such procedure and we might be wise to look at them vis-à-vis our own kinky groupings. A petition to join the Masons, for instance, includes personal information about the applicant and the signatures of three Masons who are sponsoring him. Once received, the petition is turned over to a committee of three who "investigate" the applicant, usually by visiting him in his home and interviewing him. Once this "committee" returns a favorable report, the full membership then votes on accepting the applicant into the initiation process.

Let's look at this more closely.

First, the petition contains necessary personal information to know the individual (i.e., name, address, etc.), and to verify that he meets the conditions of membership.

Second, it contains the names of three sponsors who can vouch for the applicant and recommend his acceptance into the group. The sponsors are not allowed to be on the visiting committee, thus ensuring a fairer evaluation on the committee's part. The vote taken by the full membership must be unanimous. In other organizations, a simple majority suffices.

Notice, too, that a vote to admit does not make the applicant a full member. It only allows him to begin the initiation process. Masons have three degrees through which an applicant progresses, with the idea that each degree imparts more knowledge of the group to the applicant. In the meantime the applicant is observed to insure that he is "worthy" to continue in the process.

Sound remote? The Chicago Hellfire Club (CHC), with more than thirty years' experience in membership recruitment has a very similar process. Guests are invited by full or associate members to their parties. This is how members get to know potential applicants. Only after attendance at several parties may a guest ask to join by filling out a petition.

Here, too, three CHC members (at least one full member and two associates) must recommend the guest for associate status. Upon majority vote of the full members, the guest becomes an associate, with rights and duties, but no vote. After having associate status for more than a year, an associate may, if he lives within 70 miles of Chicago, apply for full membership, though not all do so.

Such a system, either Masonic or kinky, is intended to both teach and test the applicant to ensure a right fit between applicant and members. An interesting side note about CHC membership, similar to a condition that Black Rose in Washington, D.C. has, is that full members must live in proximity to the group, insuring the new member's ability to participate fully. Full membership brings both rights and responsibilities.

Not everyone, after all, is suited for participation in every relationship. Even if the applicant is well-suited to join, there needs be a time for education, or more properly, acculturation to the customs and mores of the group. We are seeking here that the new member learn to conform to the group, not that the group be forced to conform to the new member.

I can still remember, at least vaguely, my first application to join a kinky group. I saw a classified ad to join Interchain, a gay Leather man's contact group. I sent for an application which included a very full questionnaire. Upon returning it I then had to meet a current member who would then recommend that my name be put into the quarterly directory of members.

The process echoed the practice of the rough sex crowd from the fifties: you were included because you were recommended.§ The secret

§   In the master search, references provide the same function as signers on a petition.

to joining was to find and befriend someone in the know, who would then introduce you to others, who would get to know you and eventually, you hoped, begin to include you. No one walked in and took over; no one was assumed to be ready for inclusion unless he (or she) was first evaluated.

Many professional Dominatrices have a similar process, requiring letters of application and a personal meeting before anything else transpires with their clients. In every case it is a matter of protecting the group (even groups of one) from those who would adversely affect it.

Inappropriate behavior on the part of a guest, for instance, leads to correction or an end to invitations. It is as simple as that and the system works to ensure the group continues unaffected and unharmed, while growing with the addition of new members, who learn and carry on the culture of the organization.

Notice, too, that new members are observed. Actions speak louder than words and few assumptions are made about new candidates. While strangers are welcomed and have a relative easy entrance, full acceptance into the group comes only after trial and training. Rushing untested and relatively new people into membership is frowned upon.

The Slave Petition

Lest you think that all of this is etched in stone, let me assure you that it is not. Rather than being some formal "petition" that follows the outline below, Patrick's petition to me, some nine years ago, was in the form of a letter. He told me about himself and why he wanted to become my slave. I eventually used such information to frame a contract between us, reflecting our desires for what we each wanted in the relationship.

Patrick's letter was full of facts and aptly described what he sought in a one page letter, complete with two photos and the plea that I give him a chance:

> Part of me wants to gush with excitement over having the opportunity to respond to your ad in [the magazine] Metropolitan slave. The serious side reminds me that, though you are deserving of it, you probably get that often enough as it is, and your ad was placed with more serious matters in mind. My intentions, too, are serious.
>
> Sir, I am applying for the position of slave. I am a masculine, gay, white male, with a compact 160 lbs., 5'8", average, in shape, 40 year old, moderately hairy body. I have a tight ass, uncut cock, brown balding hair when it isn't shaved, deep expectant brown eyes, and a small but hungry mouth. A stable and balanced individual, I am submissive, a bit on the quiet and shy side, eager to please and emotionally mature, with both feet (size 8) planted firmly on the ground.
>
> Sir, I am looking for a full-time, permanent master who will use me,

train, and appreciate owning a moderately experienced slave. I do not seek a lover or a Daddy, though master may choose to fill those roles. I do not seek to waste time, and though I am ready and available, I well realize the seriousness of the decisions involved. I begin this process honestly and carefully, and with great respect for the man who will be considering me. In time, a firm, caring hand can take this quality wannabe and make me into the devoted slave I wish to become.

Sir, this slave has experience in the more basic SM activities but understands that a master has the right to use a slave he owns (as opposed to a slave that makes itself available for occasional use) in whatever manner he chooses once trust is established. I know I have it in me to commit to a life of slavery. Not too long ago I uprooted myself to become the permanent slave to a master. I left a career, friends, and places with which I was familiar only to find that it was for naught four months later. Though we parted amicably, I now find myself having to choose between re-establishing myself in everyday life or continuing on, staying loose and flexible in the hope of finding that place where I think I truly belong, at the feet of the right master. As long as my finances permit, I must choose to continue my search...

Sir, you can reach me at the above address and this phone number... I know you will be discreet. I will be staying at my brother's for the Holidays and for a time afterwards before making a trip to Ohio to deal with some personal business. I will have the time to swing over to Chicago for a more personal interview should you be interested.¶

Recognizing that petitions can come in all sorts of forms, you and your applicant will have to arrive at how you want the process to unfold. I have chosen the more formal petition method because it allows us to set in writing what we've discussed and makes clear that there is the firm intention of moving ahead with the process. Difficulties, on the other hand, serve as a clear warning that our communications may not be as good as hoped and that we need to spend more time clarifying our intentions and what it is that we can agree upon.

In any case, the petition whether written or oral, short or elaborate, is meant to convey three ideas: What you want, Why you want it, and what you will give and do to get what you want.

What You Want

By this point in your dialogue, you ought to have arrived at a general idea of the meaning of slavery for each of you and the prime characteristics that you are seeking in the relationship. It's important

---

¶   This letter was received from Patrick in December, 1995.

to note that the petition need not be for anything more than a night's scene or a weekend trial run. I have asked for petitions from men who simply wanted to play — with no expectations to continue, from those who were only seeking real-time training, and from those who wanted to try slavery for a weekend, a week, or a month.

From this petition, I gain a good idea of what my applicant wants, as well as his limits and his availability. Needless to say, someone who spends time writing something like a petition is probably more serious than one who refuses.

Why You Want It

I then take the petition one step further by asking my applicant to include the why of his petition. By knowing his very personal reasons for seeking to be my slave, I have important information as to how to proceed. Is it short-term? In his heart? Simply for the experience? Later, especially during "play," I can use these reasons to reinforce the action in the dungeon or the bedroom. I will also have a better understanding of how my applicant feels.

What You Will Give and Do to Get What You Want

For my money, it's important to know that what my applicant seeks is important enough for him to be willing to offer me something in return. I am especially looking for some commitment of obedience, expressed in domestic or sexual service, or that he will give me some other form of pleasure. I then have written proof of how we will interact as master and slave. Likewise, the petition can, and often does, list protective limits and requests — made by the applicant — regarding how I will act.

The Contract

Besides serving as a milestone and clarifying event in our process, I also use the petition as the basis of a contract, so that the contract reflects not only my master/wishes, but also that which the slave-applicant seeks. Here is one that reflects my general usage:

Recognition and Acceptance of Voluntary Servitude
Dated: Month Day, Year
We, the undersigned parties, recognize and accept the submission of XXXX XXXXXXXXX, hereafter called the slave, to Jack Rinella, hereafter referred to as the Master, in a relationship of Voluntary Servitude, hereafter called "slavery." By this instrument, Master agrees to direct, train, and dominate the slave for the Master's pleasure and profit. The slave's tenure will continue for a period of one year,

beginning on the day of the signing of this agreement and ending on XXXXXXXXXXXXXXXXXXXXX .

This voluntary servitude may be renewed at the Master's discretion with the slave's consent.

It is agreed that this period of slavery will be under the Master's direction and control and will be subject to the following conditions:

Virtue will be a significant part of our relationship. Therefore, we agree that fundamental to the slavery will be the practice of the virtues of trust, honesty, openness, loyalty, and obedience. Without the practice of these virtues, there can be no true slavery. Their practice therefore is expected and required at all times.

The slave wishes to be an integral part of the Master's Leather family and will treat each person in that relationship with the respect, honor, and obedience due their position.

The slave wishes to bring the Master physical, sexual, intellectual, emotional, spiritual, and sadistic pleasure by the submission and service of himself to the Master's will. This slave will perform these things through his practice of obedience to the Master's will and compliance to the Master's rules.

The slave accepts these conditions and will strive to perform them without failure, without rebellion, and without hesitation.

For the period of his slavery, the Master will control the slave's schedule, work, education, and finances.

The slave recognizes that I, Jack Rinella, am his Master and lord and that the Master's cock is the object of his obedience and worship.

We acknowledge that this agreement binds us as Master and slave, dedicated to the accomplishment of our goals. This relationship will in no way prohibit the maintenance or development of relationships with others, except that for the duration of the slavery, the slave will make the attainment of the goals herein described his first priority and the conduct of his slavery, in light of these goals, will take precedence, when such precedence is required, over all other relationships, goals, and activities.

The slave will restrict his sexual activity to the Master and to those to whom the Master gives his permission, on an individual basis, to the slave's having sexual activity.

By our agreement to this document, the slave gives the Master the right to transfer the duties, rights, and obligations of this agreement to any person at any time for the duration of this agreement upon the condition that said person is of the same high character and trustworthiness as the Master. Those persons to whom the Master transfers these rights by gift, rental, or sale shall be deemed holding the rights of this agreement in the Master's place and shall receive the same respect, service and obedience as due the Master.

By my signature, I, Jack Rinella, accept you as my slave.

_____   Dated:_____

I, the slave, willingly submit myself to the above described slavery, commit myself to the herein described goals, and accept Jack Rinella as my Master for the duration of this slavery. By my signature, I accept you as my Master.

_____   Dated:_____

Timely Considerations

Since you've already read about my feelings regarding talking this to death, I'll try to avoid that tirade. The successful search for a master (or a slave for that matter) depends a great deal upon your readiness. The sad fact of the matter is that most applicants of both the dominant and submissive variety very often fail to be ready. On the up side of that, the process of searching itself has the happy effect of getting the seeker ready, as the process presents questions to be answered, answers to be considered, and experiences that explain and enlighten.

Ready, of course, means a great variety of things to many different people and is highly dependent upon one's personal circumstances. That consideration is compounded by the fact that we might not even know what it means to be ready. As an example, I searched for nearly eight years for a second slave and never came to the conclusion that I didn't have the necessary accommodations — namely a spare bedroom — for him. In this case, getting ready meant buying a bigger house. What then are the considerations that you need to ponder? How soon can you accomplish your goal of enslavement or submitting?

Though you may not be able to answer these questions now, you will, in time, arrive at the pressing need to answer them. The process itself will pose them and when it does, you will have to find the answer in yourself, in your situation, and with your partner to be.

How long this process actually takes is a question that only time can answer. The most critical component, of course, is how ready you are as an applicant and how confident you are in knowing what you are seeking. Added to that is the amount of effort you can honestly give to the search itself, both in terms of time and money. Once you have found a possible partner, I suggest the following timetable:

- E-mail, snail mail, and phone conversations begin the process.

- Once you seem to hit it off, the master will issue an invitation for a visit to his or her home.
- The applicant writes a petition to serve for a weekend or possibly longer.
- The master writes a contract for the duration of the first visit.
- One short visit is followed by more reflection and discussion.
- You then mutually schedule a second visit, either to your place or to the applicant's, with another contract, perhaps preceded by writing a revised petition.
- If there are indications that this is going to work out for both of you, begin to discuss living arrangements, career moves, and a realistic timetable for living together.
- The candidates spend a longer period of time together, such as two weeks or a month.
- Evaluate that visit and plan for your relocation, if that is feasible; if not, plan for another visit.
- Prior to moving in, the master sends the slave a contract which both will refine through discussion and which you both sign upon your arrival.

This process, in all likelihood, will take at least six months.

Now that I have written all this, it is important to remind you that none of this is cast in stone. For every suggestion I've given, there are exceptions, some of which don't prove the rule! Patrick has been my property for over nine years. We had one letter and two phone calls before he arrived at my door for his first visit and within a month of that visit, he moved in with me. I met Master Lynn online on a Thursday night. We chatted there for about ten minutes. He then called me on the phone. The following Saturday morning I was at his house to serve him. Two weeks later, during our second scene, he told me he wanted to collar me and did so within a month.

I am obviously very good at not following my own advice. Sometimes, though, I should. If I had, I would neither have had an alcoholic (who is none of the people otherwise mentioned in this book) move in with me, nor invited a slave-applicant who only wanted a place to crash while he attended the International Mr. Leather Contest. "Haste makes waste" is a true statement, even if "he who hesitates is lost."

The Value of Half a Loaf

Though I strongly encourage you to know what you want and to do your best to find it, it still remains a sad fact that you're most likely going to have to compromise on some of your criteria. For that reason, I strongly recommend that you remain flexible in your willingness to interview prospects and open to a wide variety of possibilities without giving up on essential requirements.

Finding a master or a slave is a process of transformation. Seeking a partner is a notice to the universe that you are willing to change (i.e., to go from being single to being part of a couple). What is less obvious is that in that transformation, you will change personally, as well. It's not just living situations here that I am discussing. There are very real psychological and emotional differences between the beginning seeker and the collared slave.

What I have found is that the search re-forms the searcher. From the day you begin learning about slavery, to the day you place your first ad, meet your first applicant, write your first petition, and so on, you will be undergoing an inner transformation.

More than that you will have to begin to reorganize your life, to some degree, letting someone else set your priorities, dictate your schedule, and control much more than simply your online play. This is, of course, a step at a time process, but a process none-the-less. If you can't obey those first early requests, how will you surrender your life to your new master?

Herein lies the value of that half loaf: it will show you in easy, non-critical ways what your future holds and whether your fantasy holds up to reality. I once had an applicant tell me that an important part of his desire to be collared was that he knew he needed someone in his life who would help rein in his out of control social schedule. He had a hard time saying no to everyone's requests and so felt like a doormat. He understood that a master could help him say no. Unfortunately, he wasn't able to surrender control of his schedule. Therefore, he continued to live as a doormat, with almost no time left for his master-applicant to ever take enough control to help him bring his schedule into a tolerable lifestyle.

All of what you have read thus far is only words. Another value to half a loaf is that it will include real-time experiences that will help you understand and more clearly define what your real goals in life are. For this reason, I encourage you to experiment with less than the "full Monty." Part-time relationships, one-scene tryouts, or a weekend spent wearing someone's collar may not be the full realization of what you seek, but it will certainly teach you a great deal more than if you had foregone the trial.

Remember, too, that there is a lot to be learned from what might appear to be a failure. Discard your fear of failure. Have the courage to try, even if it means you have to try, try, and try again. Even the applicants who don't fully conform to your dream of Mr. or Ms. Right may actually have a lot to teach you about achieving your goals. If there is a rule in all this, keep in mind that: "Nothing ventured, nothing gained."

Walking Away

By the very nature of the search, you're going to have some kind of communications with a great number of people, most of which will go nowhere quickly. It is your prerogative to choose your partner and you have a responsibility to think of yourself, and your desires first. There are lots of very valid reasons for saying, "No, thanks." You don't even have to have any more reason than a gut feeling or a desire for someone who more closely meets your criteria. It's your body, your life, and your responsibility to be your own decision maker, without any need whatsoever for apology, feelings of guilt, or explanation.

That said, there's no reason not to say goodbye gracefully, even if the vast majority of seekers will just silently and without notice stop communicating with you. If you lose interest, find someone better suited, or discover a fatal flaw, take a moment to tell your ex-applicant that you are no longer interested. It's simply good manners and also preserves the way to a second round, if and when, circumstances change and you have reason to try again.

Patrick Reflects:
Negotiation Pitfalls

There is a common belief, among wannabes and masters alike, that the master is going to perform miracles and impose behaviors that the slave could never achieve alone. Change, however, cannot easily be imposed; since it can only be encouraged, it's important as you begin this journey with your master that you make clear: the things you need and the things you think will make you better, and the steps you've already taken to reach those goals. Ask the master you are negotiating with what they've done to get ready for a slave, and between the two of you, you'll create the beginnings of a strong relationship, which gives you each what you desire. Prepare yourself and plan your journey so that you can bring worth and value to your master, so you can look him or her in the eyes and negotiate with confidence about what you have to offer.

This interconnectedness comes from the specific strengths each brings to the relationship and how each allows those strengths to enhance and complement the other. A master seeks a slave to add a special value to his life, and a slave seeks a master in order to bring a special purpose to his life. But a slave is never ONLY about the master, having no needs or insights of his own. Erotic slavery isn't about becoming a non-person; it is about becoming a more complete person. Individual strengths come together and a dance is created that allows the relationship to be fulfilling.

That's the point of negotiating: discovering the things in one another that are appreciated, discovering each other's needs, what the other wants, what is not wanted or appreciated, and the time to begin to think of how to achieve it all. It's an important process, but one that a slave-applicant often doesn't seriously consider in their determination to appear submissive or their desperation to find a master. Believe me when I tell you that how well you handle the negotiation of your relationship will determine how successful and long-lasting it will be.

Sir discusses the process fairly extensively in this chapter; so, I'll give some observations that have served me well or that I observed in watching others. I hope their value will be obvious. And while you are negotiating, use this as a checklist of sorts, if you find it useful.

It's never too soon to be honest.
This can't be said too often. The sooner you are honest, both with yourself and with those with whom you are communicating in your search, the more successful you will be.

Check your definitions.
Do you both mean the same thing when you say slavery? The time to figure that out is before you move in. Make sure your understanding of what the routine day-to-day expectations are the same as your prospective master's or mistress' — or once the newness of the relationship wears off, you'll be wondering what's gone wrong.

Communicate.
Don't sit back in awe and gratefulness that the person makes you feel the way you do, willing to ignore the little signals that could warn you of potential problems. Don't prematurely go respectfully and obediently submissive, acquiescing to any and all negotiation points. Think clearly about what they are saying and what it means for you. Ask questions, as needed, to be sure you are clear about intentions and expectations. You aren't the person's slave yet. You have the right to respectfully discuss the issues and how they would affect you.

Don't Fall Too Fast.
I've seen it happen over and over. You decide to actively explore what — up to now — you've only dreamed of and fantasized about. You take the first step in exploring and that first step touches you in ways you never imagined; so, you read it the wrong way: This must be true love! The intensity of the experience convinces you that it HAS to be

right for you and the person you are doing it with has to be THE one.

The reality is that you're drunk on new emotions. You cannot know from one encounter that this person, who has touched something deeply within, is that special person to whom you should submit forever. Later you might look back and know that was the defining moment in your relationship, but for now, be cautious. Make sure that other expectations can be as easily embraced. There's more to explore, both with that person — and with others, for comparison — before you have enough of an understanding on this new experience to know what to do with it.

You have to be true to yourself.

First and foremost you have to find contentment in order to succeed in being a slave. An unhappy relationship is neither healthy nor successful. Sometimes we have difficulty accepting the fact that even as a slave we need to be content. Voluntary servitude IS voluntary, and you can't give up your right to happiness. It's important to realize that you can and should leave a relationship that isn't providing you with contentment. Lack of contentment is unhealthy.

Don't bank on change.

Your relationship with your prospective master will succeed based on how you are (and how he or she is), not with some unrealized goal. For instance, expecting that your master will force you to get your body in shape when you've never made any progress with it on your own is unrealistic. If you aren't at least partially successful in achieving change on your own, you aren't going to do it willingly for him, even if you think you want him to force you. That kind of expectation will most likely be met with disappointment and resentment. So, be careful what you ask for. He or she is not going to change you in any major way that you haven't already established that you can change yourself.

The same holds true for your master — you aren't going to be able to change him or her. Your master may choose to change based on your influence or presence, but you can't assume or expect that it is going to happen. What if your master wants an open relationship, but you want him all to yourself? No, you aren't going to be able to change his inclinations, and attempts to try will be met with frustration and disillusionment. Don't enter a relationship with someone who holds intrinsically different values than you do unless you are very comfortable changing to meet theirs. If you can't be open and accepting of who they are AS THEY ARE then don't delude yourself into thinking you can create controlled change.

Embrace the term "wannabe" as a positive thing.

It's a way of saying "I now know what I want for myself and I have a reasonable plan for achieving it." It's far better to be a wannabe than an impostor. And it's far better to remain a wannabe than to rush into the wrong situation.

Beware of the infamous other.
Often the possibility of being a third person in a relationship comes along. If you haven't considered that this can be a good thing and the right thing for you, I encourage you to read chapter 13 and remain open to the idea, in case that possibility occurs. My relationship with Sir is the second poly relationship I've been in and I don't regret either opportunity. I think it offers much more than the traditional twosome.

With that said, beware that such a relationship is not always offered honestly. All too often, bringing in a slave as a third person in a relationship is something one person suggests to his or her partner; the partner may go along begrudgingly, or fearing that refusing would end their own relationship. If the idea is not wholeheartedly embraced by both, then the slave is going to have a rough time and the relationship will not be a "happily ever after" relationship. Two plus one only equals three if they are all positive numbers.

It's important that in negotiating any kind of poly relationship that you take extra time with each partner to discuss how the other feels about the possibility, how you will relate to each, and what each one expects from you. It's also important that each understands your expectations. All those involved need to be a part of the negotiation process. Watch very closely during the process. Are you spending significant amounts of time getting to know each of them, as well as time when all of you are together? Do you sense reservations on the part of one or the other?

All too often a slave (or submissive) is brought into a relationship because one partner has convinced the other that this new addition will bring new life to their relationship. You don't want to be a Band-Aid that is supposed to hold an unstable or unhealthy relationship together. Things will only get nasty.

Sometimes, you are the infamous other and sometimes, one or the other is perceived by their partner as being so — but either way, it does not make for a good situation. The dynamics of a threesome (or more) are far more complex than they are for a couple. Don't take the easy way out and refuse to consider a threesome. Just enter such a relationship carefully and with clear communication.

With that said, realize that you will come across relationships that are long-lived and healthy, but where each understands that because one or the other's interest and needs have changed, that it doesn't signal the end of the relationship. In that case, one partner might not be involved with the new slave, but is perfectly accepting of the other, having that enjoyment and pleasure. Being a third in a relationship doesn't necessarily mean having a significant relationship with both partners. Again, look at the situation carefully and make sure you have the opportunity for honest, individual communication with both.

If it doesn't pan out.
Sometimes, even the best possibilities are unrealized. Don't fret. There are many more potential masters out there. The search and negotiation process is merely a matter of thinning out the crowd until you find the one who is right for you. Stay confident and realize that it was both a learning experience and that you are better prepared for the next one. Don't beg or plead for it to continue, as doing so will only waste your time and the time of the master-applicant. You can always approach again at a later time, once you both have had a chance to put things in context, and have had a bit more experience looking.

Examine the process that was used.
Look at what you did to create the possibility, what you and the prospective master did to move it along, and what circumstances created the process. Use the experience to learn what could have made the process go more smoothly.

Ask for suggestions.
I mean this. Before the communication ends, ask if your applicant has any advice for you as you continue your search. Listen and don't get defensive if you don't like what you hear. Thank the person for his time and honesty think over what was said, particularly if some kind of fault with you was perceived. Then, perhaps ask a friend if the criticism is accurate.

What do you think was the reason it didn't work?
Examine the process from your vantage point. What problems or issues did you see? How did communication take place? Make notes for yourself, as that tends to give the reasons more clarity, and you will be better able to learn from the process.

What should you do differently the next time?
Move on to the next possibility, utilizing the experience you've gained and the lessons you learned.

If finding a master is a numbers game, negotiation is a mathematics problem, but this might finally be the place where you shed the label "wannabe." Think before you leap, communicate effectively, be true to yourself, and if it doesn't add up, take what you've learned and start again. Don't rush it.... Add the numbers up correctly. Any good accountant will tell you that if you go over the numbers carefully enough, they will usually finally add up.

In my own search, the most common turndown that I got was, "You're not my type." It usually was said when they received my initial letter (with photo), but it almost never involved actually meeting each other or talking on the phone. If you hear this, don't worry about it. Odds are that had the relationship been forced to develop, it would have not lasted very long. Still, it was annoying to be turned down without a serious look.

Sir and I have traveled a great deal and have met a lot of people. I've even come across some of those guys who dismissed me as not their type. As far as I can tell, they didn't remember me, but I remembered them. They were still looking for their type.

After Reading Activities

Let your fantasies run wild. Write them down in your journal. If you could negotiate any kind of relationship how would it look? Go ahead. Write down everything. Pretty impressive? Did you include all the day-to-day details? Use an asterisk to mark the qualities that you must have. Use a check mark to indicate those that are necessary, but might withstand some compromise. How do the asterisks and check marks feel? Can you live with this?

Now, write another list that is more realistic. How do you feel about this list?

List possible negatives about yourself that your prospective partner will want to know. Write how you might explain them and give reasons to him or her as to why they aren't as big a problem as they might seem.

Based on what you have learned thus far, write a sample petition Let it sit idle for three days and then go back and re-read it. Re-write it, if necessary.

Find the names of three masters whose personal ads you find attractive. Write each one a short introductory e-mail or letter, introducing yourself and asking each to consider you as a possible candidate for slavery. You might also ask your local munch, club, or BDSM friends if they know of any masters you might contact Let it sit idle for three days and then go back and re-read it. Re-write it, if necessary.

Find the names of three masters whose personal ads you find attractive. Write each one a short introductory e-mail or letter, introducing yourself and asking each to consider you as a possible candidate for slavery. You might also ask your local munch, club, or BDSM friends if they know of any masters you might contact.

5

Committing Yourself

*If you put a chain around the neck of a slave,
the other end fastens around your own.* [*]

After searching for a slave (either the first or more) for more than 20 years, I have come to the painful conclusion that all of the steps which I have so far presented are simply suggestions. None are cast in anything more permanent than the placement of pixels on the monitor displaying my word processing document.

All of the previous pages contain information which, when matched with the actual histories of men and women in real time master/slave relationships, show that the exception is more often the case than the suggestion itself. Many of my interviewees, for instance, didn't meet through any kind of ad, a few masters found slaves in the partner they already had, some have biographies that show an incredibly speedy meeting and committing. Others grew into their D/s relationships only slowly.

Whereas many masters and slaves have had mentors, most tutoring was of relatively short duration — sometimes only for the length of a single meeting or a scene. Both masters and slaves learned much of what they now know about the lifestyle through trial and error.

Many, like myself, have repeatedly entered into seemingly fruitless searches, interviews, negotiations, and even short-term relationships. Some masters, on the other hand, were led into a dominant relationship by the men or women who wanted to serve them. Go figure.

The Myth of the Plunge
Analysis of my many failures does show a frequent commonality,

___
[*] Emerson, Ralph Waldo, *Compensation Essays*, 1841.

though, that is worth considering. That thread is the "Myth of the Plunge." This phrase is a poetic way of describing the great fear of the unknown held by most submissives. In this case, fear is fed by the misconception that slavery is arrived at all at once — without hesitation, trial, or error. It is based on an unrealistic projection of the future, as if enslavement is going to happen in one great leap, as if one is "free" today and "enslaved" tomorrow. Nothing could be further from the truth.

First off, it's not really an unknown. What I have noticed is that this fear is based on that which is poorly known. With fantasies fueled by works of fiction, many subs seeking enslavement have notions that are incredibly unrealistic and sometimes patently erroneous. Though they instinctively know that fiction is not factual, they still proceed on the myth that their enslavement is going to be similar to that of Jamie (*Mr. Benson* by John Preston), Beauty (*The Claiming of Sleeping Beauty* by Anne Rice), or one of the slaves in the Marketplace series (by Laura Antoniou).

Now, this invalid thinking is often subconscious, yet operative nevertheless. Let me give an example: I recently met a guy online who thinks he wants to be a slave. As a result, his first impulse was to send me eight j-pegs of himself, in various poses of nudity and bondage. Certainly, the pictures showed an attractive candidate and I don't mean to fault him for his effort. Still, the photos conveyed the subtle idea that slavery was meant to be spent tied in ropes and leather restraints. It's not. The applicant realizes that a life of bondage is unlivable. By extension, he concludes that slavery is likewise an unattainable fantasy, when in fact it is not. Once he separates fact from fiction, he will rightly conclude that bondage is one small aspect of slavery, but not the whole part. A life in voluntary servitude is viable, while one in perpetual bondage is not.

Another example that illustrates my thoughts: I've been talking with an applicant whose last e-mail informed me that he actually dreamt we had met. It was a high power and erotic dream. After that, we talked about it and I encouraged him to make plans to visit me, an idea with which he agreed. It's two weeks later and I haven't heard a word from him since, though I have sent him e-mail and left a phone message. What's up?

I would offer that, simply put, this successful professional was overwhelmed by the prospects of quitting his job, selling his home, moving to a strange city, and serving a man he has yet to meet. His anxiety was caused by the idea of a visit, as if the visit would end with his immediately making all those changes. It won't. The visit will only be a visit, with no commitment, no promises, and no expectations, except that we get to know each other. None of the feared problems and overwhelming tasks is anywhere near to becoming a reality, even if his fantasy life tells him otherwise.

Obviously, I can only guess at the real cause for his silence until I finally get him on the phone so we can talk this through like adults. Until then, though, I might suggest that "What's up" is his fear of making a commitment, which he erroneously sees as too frightening for him to do at this point in his life. He is right, of course. It is way too soon to begin discussing long-term changes. A visit is only a visit.

Let me restate this dynamic in a different light.

The master/slave acquisition process is somewhat akin to becoming a medical doctor. Somewhere in life, a person begins thinking they want to become a doctor, which is a "call to serve." So, they embark upon the process. The call does not make one a doctor and no amount of dreaming or playing doctor will make a child, an adolescent, a teenager, or even an adult, a doctor.

One has to follow a path to doctor-hood: college prep courses, successful completion of a pre-med curriculum in college, followed by medical school, with its attendant application process and course work, followed by a difficult internship, residency, medical exams and finally, licensure. All this paves a path for the doctor to find a place to practice, when certified to do so by a medical governing board. In all, years have gone by since the first thought and the student has been remarkably changed by class work, real-time experience, reflection, and time itself.

This doctor analogy is not uncommon. Any career takes education, practice, experience, and (often) some kind of certification. Can you think of any job that doesn't include searching, interviewing, negotiation, training, and a final commitment by both employer and employee? I can't, except — of course — for a position in one's own family's business. Even then, mom and dad will have given some kind of training to their promising progeny.

Yet we labor under this unspoken myth that placing an ad will earn us a collar and then we wonder why we don't succeed. To be fair to both sides of the coupling, masters are probably no less guilty, thinking that some sex-starved 24 year old is ready, willing, and able to drop everything to wait on him or her night and day immediately, if not sooner.

I wrote, "For most of us, the quest for a partner leads to a personal ad."[†] Now, I must admit that sentence isn't quite correct. Observation shows that the reality is: "For most of us, the quest for a partner begins with a personal ad." What we are doing is jumping right into what might be more appropriately called the middle of the process. We

† See page 57.

are placing ads looking for a life changing event (becoming a slave) without defining what slavery means, understanding what it takes, or being ready to make the changes that such an event will require.

But jump in we do and then wonder why the water seems so deep and how do we keep our heads above water? Pause for a minute to read this e-mail, coincidentally received as I was writing this chapter:

> Jack, I'm not really new to the Leather scene, but I've wanted to explore more about what it's about and what it might offer me. Today I had my head ripped off by a man who accused me of being psychotic. I had answered his ad looking for a slave and I was under the impression that this was an ongoing process that required finding out our mutual needs and boundaries. When I responded to his ad, I hoped to appeal to his dominant nature by being submissive, firing up his imagination with possibilities of shaping me, but he wants a commitment with no limits and no boundaries. I backed off and he practically eviscerated me. Did I do something wrong? Is there no space for negotiation before committing oneself to someone else? Where do I go to determine if being a slave is right for me?[‡]

My reply was terse: Congratulations. You have met your first asshole who calls himself a Master... It is as simple as that. Now, what else do you want to know? Serious questions are always answered with a smile. Might I suggest you get a copy of my book, *The Compleat Slave?* Jack

I cannot emphasize enough that finding a master (or a slave) is a long-term proposition that involves incremental steps forward, slow and painstaking deliberation, and the answering of a great many questions before the collar is locked on for good and the long-term relationship is begun. It is no different than finding a spouse, changing careers, or planning for retirement. Why slave wannabes think (and fear) otherwise is beyond me.

What any review of the process readily shows is that finding that partner is in fact a dismal numbers game. It seems like the search for the proverbial needle in the haystack or the quest for the Holy Grail. I can only balance my negativity with the fact that eventually people find their partners. There are real-time humans who live the life of master and slave successfully on a daily, long-term basis. They have done so by overcoming their fears, conducting thorough searches, and persevering until they have succeeded in finding their master.

---

‡   Unpublished e-mail received November 3, 2004

Fear of Failure

Running a close second to the feeling of being overwhelmed is the fear of failure, which I will cover in more detail in chapter ten. We all experience it at some time or another. Quite frankly, we all fail once in a while, as well. Simply put, there will be innumerable dead ends, rejections, and false starts in your process — all events that will feel like failure. You will, like the reader mentioned above, meet lots of jerks, cyber-wankers, and deceivers. You will experience highs and lows, promises broken, and an incredible amount of bad manners. Statistics will bear out that I have rightly called this a needle in a haystack search.

The only way to approach the task is to keep in mind that failure is one of the best teachers, that every failure holds a clue to learning to be successful, that time is on your side as long as you are willing to make positive changes as needed and that you persevere.

There is a certain amount of risk in all of this. Risk is always with us and must be accepted as a "necessary evil." You can't avoid it. What you can do, though, is to mitigate it by taking the process slowly, being respectfully bold to ask questions whenever doubt creeps in, and to remember that we are discussing what is and always will be a human relationship.

Take, therefore, that deep breath when necessary. Pause when there is doubt to find answers to that which concerns you. Remember that your process will only be improved by experience and that "bad" experiences hold the potential to improve your process and increase your likelihood for success, just as much as the good ones do.

I cannot promise you that you will find a master or a slave. I can only remind you that "Nothing ventured; nothing gained." Like the turtle, if you don't stick your head out of the shell, you won't move ahead.

It may seem to some that my "After Reading Activities" are nothing more than writing exercises and I can't fully refute that. What I can say, though, is that they are part and parcel of journaling. This is an advantageous method that will help you think through your fears, debunk your erroneous ideas, and prepare you for meeting your potential partner. Remember that if you are a free person at this time and you want to become a slave, then you will have to change. Dealing with that change takes an important series of small steps. Eat the elephant one bite at a time. That is the only way to swallow it.

Getting Ready

What is noticeable about each and every successful master/slave partnership is that by the time it was formed, both of the partners were ready to enter into it. Readiness, then, is the one quality that you must have, even if I can't do anything more than remind you of the definition of the word ready: "Prepared or available for service or action; Mentally disposed, willing."

The sad fact is that most applicants are not ready to realize their master or slave fantasy. Think for a moment about all the reasons you are not ready: debt, career, lease or ownership of a home, family considerations, age, health, understanding of what you want, unwillingness to take a risk, unfamiliarity with the master/slave relationship, lack of experience, don't know any masters, fear, doubt, negative thinking, previous commitments, present relationships, diverting priorities, distance and geography, fear of intimacy, shame, and lack of resources.

Only you can actually list the reasons that apply to you. It is the rare slave-applicant who has no limits on their immediate availability. The best most of us can do is to move closer to a state of readiness by learning about the lifestyle, meeting prospective masters, and gradually eliminating the circumstances that prohibit our commitment to a life of voluntary servitude. In general, sincere applicants should take care to simplify their lives, without burning bridges, making no radical irreversible changes in their lives. As they say, "Don't quit your day job."

Getting ready means that one takes stock of one's present situation. Are you hampered, for instance, by onerous debt? Begin by cutting up most (not all) of your credit cards, spend only what you can afford to spend and make a conscious effort to pay off the debt. Can you afford to invest in your search? You are going to need money to travel in order to visit prospective masters. You'll find your phone bill will increase as well. You'll need substantial savings if you have to relocate, especially if you'll have to spend some time unemployed while looking for a new job.

I have had more than one wannabe admit that they couldn't even afford a bus ticket to visit me. I have responded by suggesting that they begin to put five dollars a week in an envelope as savings in order to have the necessary funds. Early in the negotiation/interviewing process, it is never advisable for one of the persons in the negotiations to pay for the travel costs of the other. Many masters, myself included, have learned that lesson the hard way, having footed the cost of the airplane ticket, only to meet a wannabe tourist, instead of a sincere applicant.

In general, quitting your job is not advisable, until you and your partner are certain that the relationship is actually going to last and any employment changes can be dealt with comfortably. On the other hand, if you are burdened with numerous material possessions, you might want to start cleaning out the attic, basement, and garage. You will, of course, want to keep heirloom items and general household goods, but stacks of old magazines, stuff that should be discarded, and items that ought to be sent to Goodwill, are all candidates for tossing, selling, or donating.

You'll also have to make plans for any pets, especially having a friend ready to pet sit when you have to travel for visits. If you are unencumbered by a pet, stay that way until you are settled in your new lifestyle.

Likewise, you will want to clear up present human relationships before you enter into slavery. If you aren't single, then you probably ought not to be looking for a master, unless your significant other is privy to the search and supportive of the possibility of having to share you with another. As a matter of fact, there are many such arrangements between consenting partners. I am only saying that you'll want to have that understanding with your partner before you get involved with another, though I will admit that cheating is nothing new, just not very productive in the long-term.

Priorities

What I am really getting at when it comes to readiness is that the sincere slave-applicant understands the importance of setting his or her priorities in order to maximize potential for becoming a slave. One could paraphrase it this way: "Priorities speak louder than words." When you prioritize your life so that your master search takes seventh or eighth place on your calendar and in your day, then your search will get you nowhere.

I am not saying that the search has to be your number one priority. I am saying that your life needs to be ordered in such a way that less important distractions take second place to becoming enthralled. You will, of course, continue to live your life in most ways as before. After all, you're still going to have to go to work, do chores, and take care of yourself. On the other hand, you don't want to mimic the slave-applicant who came to me for training and never had time to show up for the experience.

Pragmatically speaking, the productive search takes anywhere from a half-an-hour to nearly three hours a day. Look at it this way:

15 minutes	Searching through online ads, looking for a master
30 minutes	Answering those ads
15 - 60 minutes	Replying to e-mail from prospective masters
30 - 60 minutes	Talking on the phone with prospective masters plus a weekend a month traveling to meet and/or visit a master

So, you've spent anywhere from an hour-and-a-half to two hours and 45 minutes a day, plus a weekend a month of travel time, just searching.

I will be the first to admit you can spend less time and the list above will vary widely from day to day. Still, the question remains, "What are your priorities?" How badly do you want to serve? How many minutes a week will you spend working to get the new relationship you think you want?

Experience

Another important aspect of getting ready is to get experience. That's why I repeatedly emphasize that those unfamiliar with BDSM in general first join our community and learn the basics of what it is that we do. Vocabulary, mores, dress and dungeon codes, manners and protocols of a general nature, and knowledge of at least some of the fetishes that we enjoy are important foundational studies that one should complete before one decides to become a slave.

We wouldn't, for example, apply to med school before we finished grammar school, would we? Why, then, should neophytes who don't know "red right" from "yellow left," or slave from bottom, do things differently?

My own introduction to SM was a mixture of reading, discussion, and experience over a three or four year period of time. Though I didn't join a munch or club (there were none in Fort Wayne, Indiana in those "good old days"), I did meet hundreds of Leathermen, read every book and magazine I could find (there were few) and let myself experience as much of the kink as I could find.

Yes, I took risks, but they were calculated and limited. I often checked with the bartender, for instance, to make sure the guy taking me home was reliable. I spent a good amount of time negotiating the scene before it happened. I asked lots of probing questions to assure myself that my mentor for the night wasn't half-crazed or a big mouth know it all.

But I got experience for the sake of experience. Well, more precisely, I got experience because I was horny, wanted a good time, and was willing to learn. I knew, too, that experience and only experience itself would teach me what I really wanted to know.

I have tried in these pages to establish that this path to voluntary servitude is a process. As such there is no really right or wrong way to become a slave. The searching itself will transform the wannabe into a slave. Lack of action which leads to experience will only have the effect of maintaining the status quo; you'll forever remain a master-less wannabe.

Since you've read this book thus far, you are commended for that amount of seeking. On the other hand, reading alone will not bring forth the transformation you are most likely seeking. Once again, you must add action, in the form of experience, to your desires or they will forever remain just that: unfulfilled desires.

Degrees of Commitment

All of the above is meant to aid you in making the ever-present and necessary commitment. Before I continue with this section, though, it is imperative that you note that the word commitment is in lower case. Commitment is an incremental process. Rarely is it simply a matter of one big decision. Rather, it is a series of small and sometimes even subconscious choices that simply follow the path of least resistance.

There were, for instance, no weighty choices made when I loaned Steven, who was to become my first slave, a copy of *Mr. Benson*. When he agreed to read it, it was without any forethought on his part that this book would lead him into what eventually became a seven year relationship with me. Likewise, when I offered my present slave Patrick a collar, it was not a "from nowhere" decision. I had spent years (literally) studying, experimenting, and searching for a slave. Those years were filled with numerous small choices, many of which, at the time, might have seemed to have no bearing on my becoming a master, but they did.

Such, of course, is the way of human life. I had no idea, as an example, that making a sales call on *Gay Chicago Magazine* to sell them a computer would lead to my becoming a freelance writer. When I wrote my first column, I had no thought that it was the beginning of what would become my first book. When Patrick stopped at The Eagle, a Gay bar in Dallas, little did he know that decision would bring him in contact with my personal ad in search of a slave.

That is the real nature of commitment. There is seldom the need to make some grand, irreversible decision. Your choices often will be (and should be) small steps toward a goal. There will be, too, the continuing need to decide, to refine your choices, to move them slowly and incrementally towards what you now think is your goal, even as the experience of deciding and living the outcome of your decisions will expand, clarify, and change the goal itself.

Just as commitment is continuous and incremental, so too is consent. One should not expect nor give immediate and complete consent. The wiser course is that consent be progressive and expand only as our understanding of the consequences of our consent grows, combined with the degree to which we are able to trust the person to whom we are giving that consent.

Initially, then, we only consent to dialogue and even then, the dialogue often omits questions of a personal nature. No one, after all, should be freely passing out personal data to complete strangers. As our prospective master becomes more familiar, it becomes more reasonable to begin to share details of our private lives that will aid him or her in evaluating our potential. The same applies to your master applicant.

In the early stages of sharing, you don't need to know the particular details of your prospect's intimate life, especially when it comes to subjects such as finances and health. On the other hand, there will come the time, well before long-term commitments are made, that such information may not only be called for, but will be imperative. All this is a matter of gaining mutual trust over time, progressively and incrementally. Earning trust is a two-way street. You must learn to trust him or her as he or she does the same with you.

If there are no trust-building exchanges, either verbal or physical, there can be no progress in your search. It is as simple as that. Likewise, if you don't find those characteristics that encourage you to trust the other, you most likely need to address that issue directly. Without satisfactory answers to your doubts of trustworthiness, it is at best foolish to continue and at worst dangerous to do so.

Understanding the Deal

Not only is trust a necessary ingredient in creating your master/slave relationship, so is the fact that the goals and expression of your eventual relationship need to be clearly understood. Too often we let the thrill and glamour of the idea of slavery overshadow the reality of that toward which we are moving. Understanding the deal is of lesser importance when all that we are seeking is a scene, but the fact is that a long-term relationship is not a scene; it is a life-time commitment of service and mutual support.

This is why I am so adamant about the value of the written word in creating a relationship. There are many inhibitors to having a clear understanding of that to which we are agreeing and committing, and although reducing our thoughts to writing produces no guarantee that we won't fail to communicate and understand, it certainly increases the probability that our understanding the significance, obligations and benefits of the relationship will increase.

Putting your agreement in writing helps you both understand what it means, guarantees that you will remember what was agreed to, and serves as a support for the emotional and intellectual commitment you have each made.

We ought not to live our lives on unproven assumptions. By doing so, when it comes to creating a relationship, we open ourselves to the pain of misunderstanding and the eventual collapse of the relationship. Terms such as service, commitment, encouragement, support, obedience,

fidelity, submission, and the like are both beautiful and
they hardly contain any indication of the specific action:
to produce. Only by clarifying what we mean by the
grasp the implications of what we are discussing.
What kind of pleasure, for instance, do we pron
sadistic, financial, or domestic? Does it include attend
or the maintenance of squeaky-clean home? Does it mean sex ...
month or three times a night? What are the limits to sadistic pleasure
and who decides where those limits are drawn? What happens when
they are pushed and when does pushing become violating?
It is true that experience will be the best teacher as regards clarity.
A weekend together will tell more than a ten thousand word essay, to be
sure. Still once experience has indicated the meaning, it can be helpful
to render that meaning in writing against the day when our memories
either fade or our imaginations embellish the past in nostalgia.

Legal Considerations

Whereas I am an advocate of reducing our agreements to the
written word, it is just as important to remember that those papers will
have little or no legal standing. Petitions and slave contracts aren't worth
the paper you used to write them. A court of law will take little or no
part of your safe, sane, and consensual slavery into consideration when
weighing the evidence. For that reason it is imperative for us alternative
lifestylers to take advantage of the law and lawyers to ensure that we
are both protected in our relationship.

Whereas there is no legal value in our petitions and slave contracts,
there is great value in three types of properly written documents: wills,
powers of attorney, and deeds of joint ownership.

Have an attorney work with you to create these documents. They
will protect you and your partner, even if you think there is "nothing
to protect." Death, mental incapacity, serious illness, or the end of
your relationship, all pose threats to the welfare of both you and your
partner. Only the power of formal, legal documents can protect you
and your assets from disposition contrary to your will. Without them,
the state, your partner's biological family, or an angry ex can — and
very often will — lay claim to that which you think is yours.

In summary, talk to a lawyer, talk to each other, and remember that a
piece of paper will remember what you wrote a lot longer than your
mind will remember what you said.

No Escape

A common misconception about voluntary servitude, generally
promoted by those who have never been in such a relationship, is that

mes a time when ending the relationship is no longer possible. proponents of "forever slavery" fail to understand the constant nges that assault the human condition.

As in any relationship we form, the participants change over time and hence, their relationship will change. That's not to imply that change isn't necessary or that it is always bad. It just is and it always will be part of life. Change, in fact, is our only constant. So, to think that we are entering into an inescapable relationship of slavery is neither true, nor is the assumption that what we want now and how we are right now will forever remain the same. It, therefore, behooves us to plan, as part of the negotiation process, how we will modify or end the relationship, when necessary.

For the master and slave to act as if they will always be so is to be blind to reality. That's not to say that relationships can't last "until death do us part," as they most certainly can. Still, even the most rugged of relationships are bound to change over time, and wise partners will be prepared for such eventualities. In that regard, the lawyer that you consult for your wills, deeds, and power of attorneys can be most helpful.

If the fact of change isn't enough to make us mindful of the mutability of human relationships, the fact of law certainly does so as well. It is well-proven reality that "consent" cannot negate the power of law. An individual cannot give up his or her rights to safety or to change one's mind.

As an example, if you need one, the Nebraska Supreme Court, on November 12, 2004, upheld the conviction of an SM "Master" who committed five acts of criminal sadomasochistic activity. As his defense, he offered hundreds of e-mails from his "slave" seeking the activity, as well as detailing that he wanted no safe words, no possibility of release, and that if he asked to be released, it was to be denied.

[Supreme Court Justice] Stephan pointed out that the statutes regarding the non-sexual assaults make no reference to consent. An Iowa appeals court in the 1980s had ruled, "Whatever rights the defendant may enjoy regarding private sexual activity, when such activity results in the whipping or beating of another resulting in bodily injury, such rights are outweighed by the State's interest in protecting its citizens' health, safety, and moral welfare."[§]

It's obvious, then, that both parties retain the "right to leave" and for that reason, each needs to know that there is an understanding of the

§   Leonard, Arthur S., "Nebraska Supreme Court rejects appeal in prosecution of master," *Gay City News*, New York, Volume 3, Issue 347, November 18 - 24, 2004.

ending that is as clear as possible. The early stages of a relationship often cloud the future with images of bliss, joy, and "happily ever after." Still, there will be an end, even if it is decades in coming. The fact that human relationships change, and not always for the better, means that both parties should arrange for a "safety net" against unexpected tragedy. Masters should make provision for the slave's retirement, long-term health care, and financial needs, in case the relationship ends. Slaves, too, should participate in such planning so that both partners are equally protected.

Master Steve Sampson, for example, requires each of his slaves to have $10,000.00 in "escape fund" savings in order to ensure them against the day they wish their freedom from his control. To his credit, he helps them save this amount, wisely monitoring their progress for their protection. Strictly speaking, there should be no surprise in this order. It is nothing more than what any good investment counselor would suggest.

Rights

If, perchance, you were a fly on my bedroom wall or a spider perched in its web in my dungeon, you would know that in the heat of an erotic scene, I often remind Patrick that as my slave, he has no rights. Having given all of himself to me, I consider that his rights are part of his desirable package that belongs to me. They are now mine. I need no permission from him to do as I damn well please. He is mine to dominate, control, enslave, and even violate as I wish.

Ours is a consensual relationship and as such, there are limits to it, most of which Patrick entrusts to me. He can have no limits with the full assurance that my limits protect and nurture him. With that bold and necessary assurance, Patrick knows that his right to safety, to fulfillment, to happiness, indeed to living to his fullest potential is as protected by me as it would need to be by him.

Even if that weren't the case, it is legally impossible for any person to surrender all their rights to another. Doing so is impossible under the law of the land, as well as under every instinct, desire, and responsible decision a person of integrity can make. If nothing else, the right to leave is and always will be inviolable.

In view of that stark and permanent reality, my contracts have always had an ending date. Initially, they are for one year; after that I make them of two or three years' duration. The purpose of this is to allow a time, at the expiration of the contract, for there to be serious discussion as to how each of the partners have changed over the life of the contract and how those changes might affect the rewording of the contract and, more importantly, the living of it.

In fact, time has changed our contract but little. The last time we renewed it, I only asked for one change: the addition of the word sadistic in reference to the pleasure that was expected. It meant no change in practice, but affirmed my desire to explore sadism and its attendant pleasures more fully.

Having a Scene

There is probably no better indication of the potential for success (or failure) of your hoped for relationship than to actually spend some time living it. Long before the both of you arrive at words for your final petition and contract, you will want to explore and experiment with physical contact and the real experience of "doing it," whatever your fantasy life indicates that means.

Even then, as you read this chapter with the intention of becoming a full-time slave, you ought to take a moment to retreat to reality. What will it be like to spend an evening in servitude? To experience your master's touch or your mistress' caressing whip? Will you really be able to strip in her presence or don the silks that excite your master?

Unless you are far different from the overwhelming number of applicants, you will have an incredible number of scenes before you have the one where you know "This person is the One."

In practice, you will meet many masters who show promise to enslave you. Only the actual experience of submitting for a limited time will confirm the viability of that hope. That's why I can do nothing less than encourage each and every one of you to have scenes. Try out your fantasized life in small, no promises, no commitment bits. The lessons to be learned in such tryouts are invaluable. In fact, without such experimentation, you will never learn the fundamentals of being a slave.

As complete as I try to make this book, it can never substitute for real-time experience. Actually doing that of which you dream is the only way to confirm that the future you hope for is really the future that you can live. Experiencing the "life of a slave," even for two or three hours, will give you more information than hundreds of websites, dozens of books, or thousands of chats.

Any experience is better than none. Even though you will learn that the vast number of masters aren't the one you wish to serve for the rest of your life, short term experiences will speak loudly and clearly to you, guiding you to clarify and refine your objectives, giving you an improved indication of what it is you really want.

Scenes are negotiated in the same way as long-term relationships, only excluding the more personal facts that become necessary when the term becomes longer. You will want, therefore, to conduct a full interview, negotiate limits, and understand each other's expectations for the encounter. Doing so is good practice for the ultimate meeting with the one who is the One.

An important Note About Failure

Most experiments appear to fail. Scientists know this to be only too true. We master and slave-applicants need to remember that reality as well. Plain and simple statistics quickly demonstrate that the numbers game called searching for a partner has a dismal rate of return. Still, any rate above zero gives us hope that perseverance and probabilities will eventually lead us to a successful, enslaving encounter.

Nevertheless, you've got to "kiss a lot of frogs" to find that prince(ss). The only way to approach one's failure to connect is to understand two factors: one, your own inability to totally control the situation, and two, that there might be a lesson here that will lead you to improvement of the search and enthrallment.

First off, then, remember that this is a two-person encounter and therefore, half of the equation is out of your control. If your prospective isn't ready, if you are not his or her "type," if they're having a bad hair day, and if *ad infinitum*, it's just not your fault. Don't take what feels like failure or rejection personally. Chances are very high that it's nothing you did or could have done to have made it work.

We have a natural tendency to blame ourselves, when actually, no one is to blame. Take that sentence to heart and move on.

Secondly, looking on the brighter side, all encounters hold some piece of new information, or at least contain an affirmation of something we already knew. Use every "failure" as a teachable moment and find the lesson hidden in the trash heap of the encounter.

You will probably find that lesson rather quickly and easily once you get past the anger, the sense of wasted time, or the feelings of rejection. Ask yourself how and what you can learn. What can this experience teach you? What might be done differently the next time? What did you like about the encounter that reinforces your commitment to find a master? What did you dislike and why? Does what you dislike get added to your list of limits?

If self-analysis is no help, discuss the scene with an experienced player, or be bold to ask your partner from the scene to reflect with you as to how you can improve your presentation and your search. If you do discuss this with him or her, be sure to be affirming and to assure your scene partner that you are placing no blame and have no regrets, only that you want to learn from the situation so you can grow.

Part-time

Though I certainly want to encourage the formation of long-term relationships of the 24/7 variety, it is no secret that most people have commitments, responsibilities, and even desires that necessitate the creation of part-time relationships. Remember that half a loaf is better than none.

Master Lynn and I considered our master/slave relationship to be 24/7, though I usually did not live with him. Most weeks, I spent a night at his suburban-based home and on many weekends served him from Friday until Monday morning. My job necessitated that I had to be in Chicago more often than I could be at his service. I had to work outside his home in order to meet my financial responsibilities to myself and my children. Therefore, the rules and condition of my slavery were tempered by reality.

On the other hand, when Master Lynn broke his ankle and was confined to bed for several weeks, that new reality changed the way I served him; I moved in with him until he could once again resume work and no longer needed my daily ministrations. As a part-time slave, I had rules and protocols that were tailored to my schedule and the realities of our living apart.

Our agreement to become "family" to one another, and to add others to our relationship, also necessitated adaptations to our lifestyle not always found elsewhere. I was, for instance, searching for my own slave, even as I served my master. Many folks were startled by this — until they recognized the uniqueness of our (and every other) relationship.

Once again, I can only reaffirm that the relationship you co-create with your master will vary from all others. It will be shaped by your individual needs, desires, and resources. Don't let anyone tell you "how it's done," as your relationship is uniquely yours. I will venture, though, to suggest that if it varies greatly from what we generally recognize as a master/slave relationship, then you find a way to name it so that what it is you create can be clearly understood by others. A daddy/boy relationship, for instance, isn't a master/slave relationship. Please try to communicate what it is you have in a clear manner. We'll all appreciate it.

Phone and Cyber

There are many ways to co-create your relationship and it's safe to say that how you and your partner do it is up to you. Although I am not in favor of strictly virtual relationships, such as via phone or cyberspace, I'm not going to sit in judgment of you. Hey, if it works for you, that is good enough.

There are many reasons why two people maintain a virtual relationship and since this book is not about cyber-stuff, I won't go into them here. I will caution, though, that you not make more of a cyber relationship than is possible. It is only virtual and as such, lacks many of the safeguards of a physical one. Despite all assurances, you will not have the safety of body language, physical confirmation, touch, and intimate companionship to bolster your relationship. You will seldom, in fact probably never, really know that there is sincerity, honesty, and fidelity. Those cyber masters and slaves who never shake hands, look their partner in the eyes, and share a meal will never attain the quality of becoming as one.

If you can live with those limits, so be it, but don't fool yourself into thinking that the relationship will ever be anything but a pleasurable cyber chat.

I will ask, though, that you recognize that relationships ought to have a physical component, though they might not be sexual. Now this is only my humble opinion; so, please take it as that. Call your cyber master just that — a cyber master — and admit that you have a cyber relationship. Don't try and pass yourself off as what you are not. Honesty is still, after all, the best policy.

Other Kinds of Slaves

I would be remiss if I didn't mention two other forms of slavery that exist in our subculture: the guardian slave and the slave in training.

The first refers to a person who seeks a master, but has not yet found one. In lieu of a permanent master, then, another dominant agrees to mentor the slave wannabe and guide them as their master might. This relationship is also used at times when a master will be absent from the slave for a time or in the event of the master's death.

There are masters who have asked another master to look over the slave during the year following their death, usually in the form of a letter requesting that such happen. This guardianship is meant to help the slave transit back into life as a "free" person or to aid the former slave in finding a new master. It is a wise master who makes provision for his slave in the case of his own death, though certainly delegating to a guardian master might not always be necessary.

Some masters prefer to see their slaves as slaves-in-training for a period of time before they grant them the title of slave. Others take on a slave-in-training for just that purpose, recognizing that they are training a slave for service to another. There are many ways to skin a cat and many ways to create your relationship. Just remember to have fun.

113

Patrick Reflects: Making it Work

Given all of the thought and effort you have to put into the process of finding a master, you need to have confidence that this is the kind of life for you. It does no good to find someone only to find that you aren't well suited to this lifestyle. It's more than just a vague sense (or crotch sense) that slavery is right for you. It's more than the right attitude, and if you think it's about having a determination to make it work, well, it's amazing how quickly determination goes out the window when you don't like the situation you are in. This is why exploring the lifestyle is important. It will clarify your experiences and feelings, and help you focus in on what it is that you really want.

Success as a slave will depend upon other things: your confidence, good preparation, your ability to sexually arouse your dominant, your ability to be a household manager and take responsibility, finding the various ways you can serve, and your ability to be proactive in learning new skills your master will find useful, even your ability to communicate effectively and respectfully. All of these skills will take practice, and will improve with time as these tasks are the essence of what being a slave is all about. You will be more effective in some things and less effective in others, but it's not about the various bondage positions you like or how much pain you can endure.

Confidence comes from knowing you've done your homework; Now that you have found a master, there is a sense of peace that things are right in the world, and that this is where you'll prosper.

Part of the answer lies with understanding who you are and what, exactly, is a slave. Once you understand those two things, you are better able to see if service is your goal and desire.

Since you have it in you hands, I recommend finishing this book and doing the activities at the end of each chapter. Doing so will show you some things about yourself and your suitability as a slave. It's also a small test of how serious you are. If you can't be bothered putting this little bit of effort into the task, how well will you do what a future master orders you to do? In fact, once your potential master finds out you have read this book he or she will probably ask to see the answers to these activities.

Another good primer is *Training with Miss Abernathy: A Workbook for Erotic Slaves and Their Owners*¶ by Christine Abernathy. The first section will give you insights on the character and attitudes that make a successful slave, and will guide you to see how well your character, interests and attitudes match this lifestyle. They will deal with questions such as "what is a slave, what kind of slave are you, assessing your

---

¶ See Appendix D for further information on the books listed here.

strengths and weaknesses, understanding why and how this makes you feel, and determining what the risks are for you and to your everyday life, your job and family.

Another part of the answer will come from good preparation. There is a lot out there you can read, and much of it is very good stuff, but I'll list a few titles here: Sir's books, *Partners in Power: Living in Kinky Relationships*, where he talks extensively about power relationships of all kinds, and *The Compleat Slave: Creating and Living an Erotic Dominant/ submissive Lifestyle*, which is a reality-based look at how master and slave relationships work. Guy Baldwin's *SlaveCraft: Roadmaps for Erotic Servitude*, which contains advice for the slave, and *Ties That Bind: The SM/Leather/Fetish Erotic Style*, specifically the essays dealing with master/slave relationships. *The Real Thing* by William Carney is an early novel about a Top mentoring a newbie into the leather lifestyle and Vi Johnson's *To Love, To Obey, and To Serve* is the diary of an old guard slave. A book due out in early 2006 is *The Path of Service: Guideposts for Modern Consensual Slaves*, by Christina (Slavette) Parker, is a journaling workbook that will help you learn to focus and center yourself in your new lifestyle. Each of the above titles give you specific information that will be helpful in succeeding in this lifestyle.

Good preparation also includes having explored the lifestyle. You'll need to know what it feels like to have your back flogged, your tits/ nipples played with, and your crotch abused a bit. You'll need to know what it feels like to be in restraints, how leather and rope and metal feel wrapped around your body. You'll need to experience physical submission, as well as mental submission, long before you give yourself to your master or mistress for the long-term. You can do this by finding play partners, going to local parties and events, taking part in workshops offered at various regional and national events. Trust me, you'll learn a great deal about yourself and your abilities and your potential as a slave. If you leave out this key part of your preparation, you are going to have a difficult, if not impossible, road ahead of you.

You might think you want to wait and learn all of this at the hands of your future master or mistress, but that way can often create problems. There are going to be things that just don't work for you and the time to find that out is before you have given yourselves to your master or mistress. This isn't a case of mind over matter; sometimes you just can't handle a specific activity. Because we are talking about voluntary slavery, when the time comes along that your master starts to use you in a way that you really hate or can't tolerate, it's quite possible that all the work you both put into the relationship might come to a screeching halt, since **the reality is that you can say "no."** At that point, the relationship is changed, and generally, not for the better. You end up depriving your dominant of something that person really needs to fulfill his or her own desires; things just won't be the same. In essence, you had an opportunity to learn that you couldn't handle something and you didn't take advantage of it. You need to know enough about how we play to understand what you like and don't like, so that you can negotiate with your prospective master or mistress in good faith.

A key part of your success will lie in understanding what you have to offer your master and your ability to be proactive in learning new skills your master will find useful. If you are more focused on how you want your master or mistress to play with you than on how you can make their life better, then you probably won't be a very good slave. The Miss Abernathy book contains sections that discuss various kinds of tasks a slave might attempt to serve a dominant, and in the back, there is an extensive list of books — from wine selection, to packing, to letter writing, to dress and style, and many more that can enhance your ability to serve. You don't need to know everything, but once you know your dom(mes)'s lifestyle, you add to your value by your ability to adapt to it.

Another sign of a successful slave is your ability to sexually arouse your dominant. Granted, not everyone serves in the capacity of sex slave, but even so, there is still a sexual side to the relationship. Very few of you would be interested in this lifestyle if it weren't for the sex, or at least the sexual connotation of it. In those relationships where sex plays a part, your ability to arouse your master will be a key to your success. (And being REALLY good at it helps cover a lot of other sins!)

Part of that will depend on the master you find and how well you click. The fact is that some people are attracted to certain people and not attracted to others. I really don't think attraction can be determined by a photo or behind a keyboard, or even from a phone call, but many wannabe masters do it that way. In my experience, it can't be correctly determined by a brief first meeting, since more often than we realize, an attractive personality and temperament can certainly overcome any lack in physical attractiveness — if it is only given a bit of a chance. After all, your behavioral responses to different people fluctuate as situations change. Personalities vary widely among masters and mistresses and you'll find yourself appreciating some, but not others, and you will really only know that if you get to know them a little bit.

One tool of success will be your ability to be a household manager, handling responsibility proactively. Managing a household involves a lot of tasks to which you don't give conscious thought when you live by yourself, or even when you have a roommate, or live at home with family. Most things are done without thinking and there are some things you don't bother to deal with or worry about too much. That changes when you have someone to whom you must answer. You have to pay attention to things you never gave a thought to; you have to give priority to someone else's needs and desires; there will be new tasks you have to learn; and generally, there is more space and things you have to deal with. In addition, you will act as your master's right hand, doing tasks for him or her that you may not even think of now. Your ability to step in and learn how to manage these tasks is important.

Often, micro-management is the fantasy — that is, the idea of not being allowed to doing anything, other than breathing, without being told to or given permission. In a short-term scene or weekend of slavery, this kind of control might be achieved to some degree, but it's not feasible on a day-to-day, ongoing basis. Your master will have other things to focus his attention on; that can't be done if constant attention must be directed to you, following you around, telling you what to do and when to do it. It also often takes longer to tell someone how to do something and micro-manage them through it than it does to just do it yourself. The reality is that most masters and mistresses want a slave around to relieve them of mundane or everyday tasks; so, your challenge will be to take on those tasks and make them part of your routine, turning the mundane into opportunities to serve. Don't be the kind of slave that has to be micro-managed all of the time, though every master will have their own little things they like to control in detail. You'll be of far more value to your master if you learn what is expected of you and when it is expected.

You'll discover the best ways you can serve and your strong talents in the first several months into the relationship. You won't know them right off, and a lot of the knowing will only come naturally as you adapt your ways to those of your master. This adapting takes up a lot of energy and focus. Your master, too, will have new skills and talents he or she will expect of you and you will be putting energy into being successful in those new ways of service, as well.

There will come a time when you are fairly comfortable and secure in your service. Things will become routine, and after a while, you'll start getting a bit bored or restless in your role as slave. That's when it's time to be proactive, to develop new skills that will be helpful to you in your service or helpful to your master. It's akin to taking on a new hobby and, lest this start to take the focus off of your master or mistress, look for "hobbies" that will also be beneficial to the relationship and your service to your dom(me). You might even create a list of things that would be both interesting and beneficial, and then discuss them with your master or mistress.

New skills can take on a variety of interests: learning about wine, learning more efficient ways to pack luggage (really!... there are helpful books on the subject.), learning about opera or jazz (as opposed to just listening to it), the art of entertaining, gourmet cooking, letter writing, valet service, organizational skills, sports; most anything that is of interest to your master or mistress will have resources available that will allow you to learn more about it. The more you know, the more complete your service can be.

For instance, Sir seldom complained about what I fixed him for meals. When I moved in, he was eating out of cans and boxes; so most anything I put more time into preparing was an improvement (though he still insists that I keep an ample supply of canned ravioli and canned beef stew in the pantry) but I was still a fairly basic and untried cook. Previously, I either lived by myself or lived with someone who did most of the cooking; so, there wasn't much energy put into learning to cook more than simple meals. I found I enjoyed cooking; so, I took on the task of improving my skill and being more creative with the meal menu. It improved even more when our friend, John, became Master Lynn's slave. There were many times I would consult with John on how to do something and many cooking tips he showed me. Even when he didn't know, he would help me find out. John passed away last year, and even though I learned a great many things from him, there are still times when I wish I could pick up the phone and double-check something with him. He is sorely missed.

This reminds me that another necessity for succeeding as a slave is help. Do you really want to thrive as a slave? Meet other slaves with whom you can be friends to some degree. They will be excellent sounding boards and their advice will take you far. Good slavery doesn't happen in solitude.

Cooking is often part and parcel of a slave's responsibilities, but there are many more interests you can take on to improve your service skills. The *Training with Miss Abernathy* book has a very lengthy list of suggestions and resources that you should check out. You'll find many interesting and beneficial things that will enhance your service to your master or mistress, and hence your value to them. It will also help keep your slavery from getting too routine or boring.

Your ability to communicate effectively and respectfully with your master or mistress is perhaps the single most important skill you should — well — master. Far too often, Sir comes across slave-applicants who haven't been successful in finding or keeping a master, simply because they haven't learned to communicate effectively. Communication will increase your ability to understand your master or mistress and what is expected of you.

Effective communication involves learning to listen, as well as learning to express your thoughts and feelings. All too often, in an attempt to be more surrendered and slave-like, submissives adopt silence or "quiet" as a way of expressing their submissiveness. Many will go so far as to be compliant and passive and end up being too much so. This evolves into not communicating your needs or feelings, until they reach the point of frustration. I often say "I'm submissive, not stupid," but slaves all too often encourage the perception that they are incapable or not able to handle responsibility, or make decisions by not communicating effectively. In our quest to remove ourselves from the center of attention, we end up right back there again because we fail to communicate well and it begins to create problems. If you are going to succeed as a slave, take steps to improve your communication skills. Find a good book on communication and learn from it. It will be well worth your time.

Two good books on communication are *Messages: The Communication Skills Book* by Matthew McKay, and *Getting the Love You Want* by Harville Hendrix.

After Reading Activities

Use your journal to make a list of things that you fear can go wrong in your search for a master or that might happen once you are enslaved. Write this list freely, either on paper or in your mind, without editing it. Let it sit for a day or two, re-read it, and add anything that might have since come to mind.

Now look closer at this "fear list." How realistic is it? Rate each fear as serious, only lingering, or completely unrealistic. Label each fear as controllable, not worth thinking about, or needs to be addressed. How will you "control" the controllable fears and what might you do with the ones that need work?

Keep a diary for a week that notes how you spend your time. After the week is up, analyze how our time is spent and consider how much "free" time you have to do your searching and your learning. How can you adjust your priorities so that you can find your master or mistress sooner rather than later?

Consider what experiences you lack in various BDSM activities, such as flogging, bondage, or D/s protocols. What skills might you need to learn in order to become a better slave, such as housekeeping or cooking? How can you learn these common or kinky activities? Who might teach you? Develop a plan to improve yourself by gaining experience. Review the plan on the first of each month to see if in fact you are working to reach your goals.

6

The Training Process

However wise you may be already, on this Path you have much to learn; so much that here also there must be discrimination, and you must think carefully what is worth learning. All knowledge is useful, and one day you will have all knowledge; but while you have only part, take care that it is the most useful part.[*]

One of the more valuable undertakings in the pursuit of the best SM is to learn about it in whatever way one can. Knowledge, in this regard, empowers us to enjoy our kink to the utmost and to discover and express ourselves to the fullest extent possible. Learning is an imperative ingredient for human growth and if we can learn from others, then our learning curve will be accelerated.

Education takes on a great many forms: experimentation, study, practice, listening, and discussion are examples that quickly come to mind. Though we most often think of "training" as something that applies mostly to the master/slave or the handler/puppy dynamic, in fact it can be an important part of any person's education in kink, no matter what the subject.

My handy American Heritage Dictionary defines the verb "train" as: "To coach in or accustom to a mode of behavior or performance; To make proficient with specialized instruction and practice." The best SM experiences come with being proficient: "Performing in a given art, skill, or branch of learning with expert correctness and facility; adept."

Though my slave, Patrick, has only a few protocols that I require of him, one of the ones performed most often is when he greets me.

---

[*] Krishnamurti, *At the Feet of the Master*, Yogi Publication Society, Chicago,

Upon our meeting, such as when he returns from work or I come back from school, he will drop to his knees and kiss each of my feet, then recite a required phrase. Though the action has been required since the beginning of our relationship, the phrase has changed over time. Originally, I think, he said "I was born to serve you," then I changed it to "I live to suck your cock." There were several others that I can't recall. The present one, "Please train me to please you, Sir," evolved a few years ago.

When my fourth "second" slave left, I decided that if I couldn't have two slaves, I would make one slave give me the pleasure of two. "More slavery, Patrick," I would say. "I want more slaves and more slavery." This led to the idea that if he was to become more of a slave, I would have to train him in specific areas of service. If I wanted a more intense relationship and more intense experiences, then I would have to lead him there with me.

Over the next nine months or so, then, I incorporated "training" into our sex life. Let's see. I have trained his lips, cock, nuts, and ass. We have had training with ropes, belts, paddles, crops, dildoes and clothespins (one of my favorite) and have trained for pain, endurance, control, and my pleasure.

Novices often fail to understand that more experienced players got there through experience, direction, and practice. I remember the first time I heard of someone getting fisted. I thought that such a thing would be impossible. Indeed, if you have a virgin ass, it isn't easy or even probable that it will get penetrated by a fist quickly. Only later did I realize that the sphincter muscles can be trained to relax so as to become open enough to accommodate a fist. That process, like all training, is done in stages, with the number of the fingers or the size of the dildo inserted increasing only with time and practice. Small steps, folks, small steps.

One learns, for instance, to tolerate one clothespin, then a second. In this way tolerance of the pain is gradually learned. When Patrick first submitted to me more than nine years ago, he was, for instance, quite adverse to my slapping his face. The first time I did it, I got a strong, angry reaction. I had tapped into a significant amount of fear.

Eventually he learned to take my hand on his cheek. In early 2004, I began "slap training" him in earnest. When I train, I make known the goal of the training; so, I began by saying something like "Patrick, you need some slap training and I'm going to give it to you." I tell him what I want and why I want it. I then build the intensity of my slaps slowly, during which time I will reassure him that I won't hurt him. There is a great deal of reinforcement that must take place, as well.

I especially want him to know how much I enjoy slapping him, as my pleasure is a big concern to him. I acknowledge how much he has improved over time with practice and what a good slave he is to have learned this and to have learned it well. This procedure applies to any SM practice in which one wants to become proficient. It is a matter of setting a goal and creating a plan that will lead to proficiency. The plan should incorporate positive feedback in order to reinforce the desired behavior.

Look for training, then, that rewards more than it punishes, that affirms and empowers rather than puts down and shames. How your training is conducted will tell you as much as what the training entails. The quality of the instruction reveals the quality of the teacher as well. Look for practical instruction and positive reinforcement.

Behavior sets real SM apart from fantasy and cyberspace. Actions speak louder than words. Are you a top? Then show me your dominance in your behavior, not your attitude. If you are a slave, then behave as such. No amount of talking, and there can be a lot of it, is as credible as behavior that is witnessed. If you tell me you really want something, such as a partner or to know how to use single-tail whips, then let me see the behavior that demonstrates your desire and makes it believable.

This applies to all of us at every level of our Leather life. Training is invaluable, if we are to gain the proficiency needed for the fullest expression and enjoyment of our kinky lives. Unfortunately we too often fail to understand that much of what is good in SM demands training. In this era of rapid gratification we just want our ecstasy to be handed to us without effort.

Too often, too, we let other considerations interfere with the realization of actual learning. For instance, we might refuse to learn from someone who is the "wrong" age or weight or gender. Training, you see, can come from anyone who has the necessary skills to transfer the information to you and will help you gain the experiences you need to become experienced. We need to get over the expectations, self-imposed requirements, and hang-ups that deter us from attaining our goal — having enough experience to become a slave.

I know that all this sounds like work. It is. On this planet, little comes easily so it behooves us to be willing to "pay the price" in order to grow as Leatherfolk. What then do you want to be different in your kinky life?

Make a list. Doing so is a behavior. Prioritize the list, as you can't have it all at once. Are there some things that can be acquired easily? Do them first as you make plans and work toward the more difficult or more time-consuming objectives. Write out your plan and give it substance with dates and bench-marks for determining your success.

Review your plans and revise them as necessary. Do you need

training? In what area? Where can you find someone to help you? Are you willing to do what it takes? The answer to those questions will only be proven by your actions. Remember it's only a series of small steps. Take care to do the small steps and the large ones will happen with your hardly noticing.

Unfortunately, Leatherfolk often use the word "training" euphemistically. They're really talking about having sex, not getting an education. So, masters advertise that they will train and slave wannabes go looking for the same thing. That's not to say that our subculture doesn't do a lot of real training, since it does — but one-on-one training can often just be play. Good mentoring is more than just play, though play may certainly be part of it.

On the other hand, there are a multitude of kinky environments that allow for training: seminars, weekend retreats, demonstrations, and just watching the action around us, all teach us something. What though does real training encompass?

Over the years, I have volunteered to train many people and I can honestly say that the process has never lasted very long. In truth, I think that's because the training was successful. It taught them that they didn't want to be slaves. For some, that is an important lesson.

In this chapter, I am discussing more generalized training, such as learning the general mores and customs of our lifestyle and gaining a familiarity with the broad range of activities common to most master/slave relationships. In the next chapter I will try to focus on the more specific and couple-determined characteristics that the slave will need to know.

We often think that training means that we learn how to perform a specific function, which is certainly true, but along with the training, we can gain significant insight into ourselves, our motives, and our true desires. Limits, for instance, can be pushed to the point where one or the other says, "Stop." Often thought of as failure, such a request actually says, "I've discovered this is past my limit." That's not a bad thing to know.

What are the aspects of training that we might consider? I would list them as introduction, direction, explanation, performance, evaluation, correction, and repetition. Allow me to examine each of these. First you also have know what it is you want to learn.

Defining Goals

I am writing this book with a clearly stated goal: "In short, this book is about change."[†] For me, that means that this book will help you become

---

† Page 5.

a slave. Stated otherwise this book is about creating slaves.

What are your personal goals and how do you define them? What goals does your prospective master or slave have? Which goals are the same, which complementary, and which pose difficulty?

Pedagogically, if we are to have a successful training process, we need to know the goals that the training is to accomplish. After all, if you don't know where you are going, you're not going to know when you've arrived. Knowing your destination allows you to plan the trip, collect the necessary resources, and make intelligent choices among a wide variety of possibilities.

Unfortunately, some people just meander through life reacting to it, rather than trying to be proactive. They have no long-term goals because they haven't taken the time to know themselves, what they truly want, and how they want their lives to unfold in the next five, ten, or twenty years. The result is that some five or ten years later they are still adrift, buffeted by life's circumstances and still hoping for the best, without any plan for attaining it.

Good training has a goal. It is as simple as that; so, start with your goals. Yes, they will change over time, but still they will provide necessary guideposts for your decisions and your success.

Introduction

Though it may be the shortest of the steps involved in training, it is important to introduce the topic to the student, if only so that he or she may know that what is going to happen next is, in fact, meant to be learned. The introduction focuses the mind on the directions that follow and differentiates the actual training from play. It boils down to some kind of "listen up and learn this" and may be as simple as those five words.

Direction

It then behooves the instructor to give clear directions as to what is to be learned. This is the what of training: Do such and such this way or first do this and then do that. The degree of specificity in the instructions will vary, depending upon the learner's knowledge of the subject and his experiences with the activity. It may, for instance, be as basic as saying, "Bring me orange juice every morning," or as complex as explaining how to cook a turkey, balance a checkbook, or run a computer program. Training for sexual activity is, of course, going to include a great many specific instructions regarding position, attitude, preparation, execution, and pre- and post-cleaning.

One premise here should not be overlooked. I believe that it is the responsibility of the teacher to ensure that the student understands the instructions. To give unclear direction is to set the student up to fail. Likewise, it falls upon the student to realize the important role they have in asking questions and giving feedback to their teachers.

Education is always a two-way street. Passivity in training will only slow down the effort. Yes, you may be a submissive, but that in no way implies that you are non-responsive, or that you can be non-involved. Look, too, for trainers who understand this reality, as they make the best teachers.

Explanation

Concurrent with, or immediately following, the giving of direction, it's helpful to give the why of the lesson. Again, this may be as simple as saying, "Because it makes me feel good," or more complex, depending upon the request. In any case, our instruction should be holistic, satisfying not just the physical person, but his intellectual and emotional sides, as well.

This advice is occasionally contrary to practice. Some tops like to keep their bottoms in the dark. I am personally opposed to such tactics, as I strongly believe in the necessity of full disclosure and good communication. Now, if all you are doing is playing games, then it's less of a problem. If that is the case, of course, then you're probably not really interested in true learning.

Performance

OK, you've laid out what you want done. So, now it's time for the student to do it. Talk without action is useless. In fact, performance itself is often the most important part of the training process, as we often learn best by doing.

Evaluation

Having performed, so to speak, then there is the need to evaluate. Was it done correctly? Did it point up other areas where training is needed? Is there the necessity for more practice or better explanation? Indeed, the training process demands a great deal of feedback in order to be successful. It may occur by observation or by examination, but either way, it should be done to lead into correction, if necessary, and eventually, to positive feedback that reinforces the desired outcome.

Correction

Correction may be as simple as further instruction or may include punishment. Certainly, positive reinforcement is to be preferred, but punishment has its place, as well. I need to qualify the sentence with the notion that punishment must be judicious. When I train, for instance, I begin with direction. If the directions aren't followed, I give further instruction. If that isn't effective, I then give warning that further poor performance will be punished. It is important to punish only when the punishment is expected. I punish for disobedience, not mistakes.

When I taught Patrick to play with my tits as he sucked my cock, for example, I first told him what I wanted. When he failed to remember to do it, I would count out loud as a reminder. When counting failed to produce the desired effect (his hands on my tits) then I warned him that if I had to count again, he would be punished. Punishment, in this kind of situation, works well. I will discuss this more fully in chapter nine.

Repetition

The last part of training is repetition, as practice makes perfect. Repetition also allows for gradual increase in intensity and improved dexterity.

Of course, most training of the formal kind doesn't present the opportunity for all of the above, especially punishment. I can't exactly give a lecture, followed by a written test and administer punishment when my audience fails. For the most part, our training is going to be demonstration and explanation. In the usual scheme of things, the learning process is really left more to the learner than to the trainer. In master/slave training, though, and to a lesser extent in Daddy/boy relationships, the training can more closely follow the above outline.

As I reflect on this chapter, I am very mindful of the necessity of good training in all we do. We take such an idea for granted when we consider flogging, bondage, or fisting, but it applies just as much to manners, organizational procedures, and decorum in meetings and dungeons. It is up to all of us to remember that we are all teachers, especially by the example that we give to those around us.

I need, too, to reinforce the importance of evaluation, lest it be seen as simply a process where the teacher evaluates the student. In fact, we must continually evaluate the lessons that SM brings to us. Doing so allows us to more deeply understand ourselves, our needs, and our motivations. Good evaluation of self, the process, and the experience will teach us much and steadily improve the pleasure and the fulfillment that a kinky life offers. Teachers, as well as students, need to be evaluated, thereby giving all the chance to learn.

It is easy enough to see our kinky play as merely diversion. For many, that might be the case. Real leather, I think, probes more deeply and brings greater pleasure by fostering an atmosphere and opportunity to learn and grow.

Encouragement and Inspiration

In all of our relationships, it is important to encourage and inspire our present and potential associates. This especially applies in the training process. There is no doubt that positive reinforcement is highly effective and carries much less risk than does negative reinforcement (punishment).

For that reason, for example, even as we are flogging the hell out of a bottom's back, we take time to caress and kiss them and to tell them what a good job they are doing. Just as this feedback does much to make the scene soar higher and last longer, so too do the "atta boys" and "well dones" given during slave training, have a highly positive effect.

Humans have incredible potential. Inspiration, then, is encouragement to reach this potential. That's why I have included explanation and rationale as an important ingredient in the successful training process.

Why include all of this in a book about becoming a slave? I do so because a fuller knowledge of the process will not only help the trainer, but the student, too. Better understanding of the dynamic of training will not only encourage and inspire you, but will also serve as an excellent guide in your choice of a master or mentor. Choosing your teachers well, after all, is one of the ways to ensure you get a good education.

That's not to say that good teaching methodology is the only criterion you need in a potential master. In fact, your master may not be a teacher at all. Still, there will be many teachers in your life and recognizing the good ones can be very helpful. On the other hand, there is no way I can know what your process, your education will be like. So, don't get too hung up on any one pattern or procedure. Instead, look for that which both feels right to you and which leads to success.

Removing Blocks and Unloading Baggage

I could title this section in many ways, depending upon the slant I wanted to give my thoughts. Since a reader named Sherri once quoted a column I wrote about being "freed from the constraints of emotional and psychological baggage," the title I've chosen seems appropriate.

She went on to ask "Is that actually possible?... While I would love nothing more than to escape from all of life's demands and 'find' myself, that is a fantasy. The reality is I have commitments, responsibilities, and any escaping I do, will have to be accomplished within those boundaries. Nevertheless, I would like to get past the illusions of who I 'ought' to be. How does one do that? How does one change their mindset to a place that's so different from all they've known? I was raised to respect, obey, and conform. Now, in my 30s, I'm discovering a rebellious streak. Doesn't seem to make much sense. Yet, I find myself fighting to continue the discovery process. Where do we dump the baggage and how?"

There is no short and easy answer to Sherri's question. I will note that chapter five of my book, "Partners in Power," covers the question in about twenty pages. That's nowhere near enough for a complete answer, but it's a start and I hope, a good one.

That said, I will say that the short non-answer is to get experience. Knowing, accepting, loving, and understanding ourselves is all part of a process, which I believe explains the why of our existence. We are here to learn about ourselves and to find the courage to be that self.

Without experience, we can have no knowledge. In this context, I would clarify my words by noting that experience is of the "experimental" type. I am not advocating jumping off cliffs or going whole hog. Let small safe experiments in Leather give you an indication of what can be. Whether that indication is positive or negative, it is a valid learning experience from which you can grow.

Note, please, that failure can be a very positive experience. Edison, as the story goes, discovered a thousand ways not to create a light bulb. It was on the basis of those failures that he learned how to succeed. That illustrates the first principle. Try it and see what you learn. Is being freed from blocks and baggage possible? I really don't know for certain. I hope that death frees us from our constraints, but I have no proof of that as of yet.

My questioner quickly moved from freedom to escape, a leap that I am not willing to make. There is no escaping. There is only growth or decline, knowledge or ignorance, betterment or deterioration. Boundaries are not necessarily bad things. My skin is a kind of boundary for my body and I'm not ready to jump out of it, though that is not a totally unpleasant thought.

How does one get past the illusion of what one ought to be? By learning that those illusionary constraints are just that and accepting real boundaries, as existent, as well. To be frank about it, this takes courage. I fear (and hope that I am wrong) that most people don't have the courage it takes to chose freedom. They seek the illusionary comfort of the status quo, the approval of others over their own happiness. They have lost their creative ability to look outside their world view, beyond their past. I must admit to my pessimism here: I think most people are unhappy.

Getting beyond those "oughts" takes time. You need to know them first, then be able to discern which ones to keep and which to change. Understand from whence they came and why. Analyze them historically, socially, legally, physically and decide which are valid for you, which are helpful, and which are better discarded.

In all of this, the benchmark is your own heart. There are two tales that come to mind here. The first is of a man who fantasizes about a life of bondage, chained or caged forever by a top who assumes all control, all responsibility. At present, he spends hours, even days, watching videos of SM activity, masturbating over and over again with the fantasy of it all. Then, his sexual passion wanes and he gives up on the idea, only to return to it when his hormones drag him there again. He is trapped by fantasy and paralyzed by his lack of knowledge and courage. His only information is what he sees on the video. There is no community to support and sustain his growth, no understanding of how to separate fact from fiction. When I once told him that I was going to Kansas City to speak, he was dumbfounded, disbelieving that there could be a group of like-minded kinky people in Kansas. Turn off the VCR, guy, and get real experience.

The other tale is more heart-warming. A young man named Eddie came to me more than four years ago seeking to be my slave. For four-and-a-half months we met, talked, and played. If you go back to the columns I wrote during that period, you will find a roller coaster of emotion, doubt, and fear, fed by his right-wing, fundamentalist family.

After those four-and-a-half months, I saw Eddie only rarely, as that was his choice. Since the days of our playing, he has learned a lot about himself. It took courage. He had to face his fear of loss, and make a choice that living his life in his way would be better than living it in his parents' way. He had to decide what to believe and why. Then, having done so, act on his faith. Action is the necessary ingredient here because "Faith," as our Christian friends say, "without works is dead."

Years later, I ran into Eddie at the Cell Block, one of our local Leather bars. He was a completely changed individual. Happy, vibrant, self-assured, positive about his gayness, in a relationship that he obviously enjoyed. He filled my heart with joy by just being himself. He said, "Jack, you were right. It only took time."

Yes, time heals while it teaches. In the midst of the trauma, though, it never feels like time passes quickly enough, unless, of course, it feels like it's passing too quickly. Acts bring the experiences that inform faith, that instill knowledge.

I was turned on nearly twenty years ago by those same videos that I mentioned above. I jerked off to them, as well. I wasn't content, though, to merely masturbate my desires into a cum rag. I had to meet those people, or at least meet people like them. I had to ask them questions, watch them play. I had to feel the ropes, the crops, the floggers, and the leathers. I had to get real experiences that would tell me "This is good," or "Avoid this."

I think I knew even then that it took courage. I was often afraid as I walked into yet another dingy Leather bar on some dark, alky-infested street. I only knew there was a hunger within me that demanded to be fed, to be understood, and to be satiated. Empirical knowledge, first gained though reading magazines and books, through watching videos, then by meeting real people who shook my hand, shared a beer and told me their stories, was the key. From there, I went home with them for the experience. To feel their piss on my stomach, their ropes in my hands. To spank them and see how it felt and let them give me the same pain/pleasure. Experience added to experience, and as Eddie said, time taught well.

This book is about change, which leads to the unknown. Facing the unknown takes courage, but take heart as you can change into that which you seek.

Panic and Prevention

Before you get the wrong idea, the subject of this section, like many of the "dangers" of BDSM is not widespread. Yes, panic happens but not as often, and certainly not as seriously, as your paranoia would make it seem.

Panic is one of the things that can happen during play. It is as simple as that. Likewise, it is one of those things that can be prevented, solved, and passed through, without necessarily ruining your play. Of course, it must be understood and dealt with. Most importantly, it should be prevented. Let's see how all this works in real life.

My trusty American Heritage Dictionary defines panic as: "a sudden, overpowering terror, often affecting many people at once." Terror, then, is: "intense, overpowering fear," and fear is: "an emotion of alarm and agitation caused by the expectation or realization of danger."

Analyzing those definitions, we see that fundamentally, panic is an emotion directly related to some kind of danger. In our case, we can probably weigh more heavily on the word "expectation," though there are certainly times, albeit they be few, that the realization of danger may be actual. In truth, the fear is most often illusionary, but that doesn't necessarily make the emotion any less overpowering or intense.

There are, it seems to me, three ways to look at panic: from the view of the top, of the bottom, and as regards its prevention.

Prevention is the best cure for panic, involving both communication and preparedness. Communication before the scene builds trust and establishes limits. Headspace, where your head is at, is crucial to the progress (or regression) of a scene. If either of you is in a poor headspace, then you are, in fact, prime targets for a less than pleasant scene. We negotiate in order to put ourselves into a headspace where mutual trust and understanding are assured. That's why good negotiation is so very important. Where there is the bond of trust, fear will have less power to encroach upon our fun. On the other hand, poor communication will foster fear.

I would add that this involves the communication of one's feelings before the scene. The declaration of illness, fatigue, moodiness, anxiety, repressed anger, or even "a bad day at work" can be effective means of changing the dynamic of the scene for the better, because potential problems will be more easily noted and thereby, the players will be better prepared to face them. The other part of prevention is preparedness. (How's that for effective alliteration?) Though good preparation may seem to be one person's responsibility, it is, in fact, the task of both partners. Just because it's my house or my dungeon or the responsibility has been delegated to one person (i.e., "Get the playroom ready boy. I'm horny"), doesn't remove the responsibility for being prepared from the shoulders of the other. Safety is, and always will be, a mutual (equally shared) responsibility.

What it means to be prepared is highly specific, depending upon the kind of scene you're going to have. Mummification, for instance, means that you know where the scissors are so you can cut the bindings quickly, if necessary. Bondage in chains, on the other hand, would have no use for scissors, but quick release snaps and bolt cutters are very appropriate.

Good training, too, is a critical component of preparedness. If you don't know what you're doing, get taught before you try. Knowing that both you and your partner are prepared will do much to prevent the emotion of fear from rearing its ugly head. Know, too, the techniques that overcome panic: quick action, quick assurance, soft words, and gentle touches.

The Bottom's Responsibility

On the bottom's side (where panic is most likely to start) it is important to keep the top informed of the feelings that the scene is generating. Speak up and let your top know what emotions are flooding your brain. Don't expect him or her to be a mind-reader. If you feel anxious, if danger seems near, let the top know, so he or she can deal with it before it becomes a serious problem.

Silence on the bottom's part is a dangerous thing, as it will easily mislead the top into a false sense of security. Remember that you both have a responsibility to ensure safety and that means that the submissive must do what is necessary to aid the top in achieving that goal.

For the Top

From the top's side (and tops can panic too), it's important to remain in control of oneself and not let the bottom's panic, or your own, take over the scene. Often, the mere acknowledgment of the condition is the beginning of the cure. It may be as simple as saying, "I understand there's a problem. Don't panic. I'm taking care of it," as you do, in fact, cut them loose or whatever it takes to remove the appearance of danger.

Reminding the bottom of what to do is an important remedy to the problem of panic. During one of my first scenes with a slave-applicant he panicked because of his fear of being fully restrained. In fact, it was a position he had wanted me to put him into. When he got what he wanted, it was, at the time, more than he could handle. It fell to me then, to remind him to relax, to breathe, and to surrender. I had to tell him he could trust me and that I was attending to the problem by releasing him. His panic soon past, but I released him nevertheless, so that we could discuss what had happened and I could teach him how to handle the situation. What he perceived as a failure was turned into a learning session, one that we haven't needed to repeat.

The emotions of one of the players will increase or lessen the emotions of the other. Hence a soft word will disarm a harsh one. A gentle touch will help overcome thrusts and gestures of panic. At times, of course, one must be a bit more controlling, holding the one who is panicking so that the solution can be administered.

My rule is that panic always stops the scene for the moment. When there is that amount of fear present, I am certain it's time to take a break from the action. The break seldom ends the scene entirely, but does interrupt it so that we both have time to bring our emotions under control and, if necessary, to understand what just happened.

With new partners, the scene may, in fact, have to end. With long-term partners, it may be as simple as taking that break and then moving into a different activity. There's even the possibility that once the panic is acknowledged, the scene can continue, but that evaluation must be made at the time, never assumed.

As I said when I began, panic is not a prevalent problem. Still, that ounce of prevention is well worth the price.

In Summary

Learning is a life-long process and comes from many sources. Prior to meeting your master or mistress, there are numerous things that you can and ought to learn. This allows you to arrive at the dom(me)'s feet with a clear understanding of yourself, and the general expectations of what constitutes a life of kink, combined with one of obedience and service.

Still, there are no actual qualifications needed to begin the search, except the desire to do so. Once begun, you will learn what is required and will either meet those requirements, or change your expectations. Most, of course, cease to search, wisely understanding that voluntary servitude is a calling not for the faint of heart or for those who merely seek thrills, sex, or escape. As in becoming proficient, in any career, slavery will make demands on your time, energy, priorities, and commitments.

Learning to become a slave will change the way you act, think, and hope. Your ideas will be challenged, reformed, clarified, debunked, and repeatedly tested. You will undergo a long, arduous process that will eventually lead you, if you persevere and are willing to change, to finally kneel at your master's feet. It is then, remarkably, that your real training, that which moves from the general to the particular, will begin.

Patrick Reflects:
Real Training Isn't What You Think It Is

It seems to me that far too many, in searching for a master, haven't done the important work of discovering just what "slave training" is. They jump over being a wannabe and claim the "title" of slave long before they know what expectations come with the title.

I've read the ads and seen some of the e-mails Sir gets. A common request is "to be trained as a slave." I've always been a bit puzzled by that because I'm not sure, at least with some that have visited Sir, if they really knew what it was that they were requesting. It isn't a "one size fits all" kind of thing. Usually they have little clue what being a slave is all about. I got the impression that when they left, they really didn't find what they had asked for.

After so many e-mails, I've come to the conclusion that, more often than not, they requested one thing, when they were really looking for something else. Not that Sir didn't give them what they said they asked for; they didn't understand the lifestyle well enough to ask for the right thing. Many seemed amazed, for one thing, that the pleasure and attention was focused on Sir rather than on them. Others seemed unhappy that they weren't put into heavy bondage scenes for long hours. Some seem very surprised when they realized that Sir expected them to help around the house, like cleaning up from dinner, or cleaning the bathroom.

In my experience, "slave training" is something that occurs once you have been claimed by/given yourself to a master, and it is the process of learning the things that bring pleasure to your Master, in the way he prefers, rather than having pleasurable things done to you. The next chapter will talk more about being trained as a slave, but before you turn there, I want to dispel some other misconceptions about training.

It starts sooner than you realize. While today there are workshops and seminars[‡] on the subject, there was no "Acme Slave Training Service" that I knew of back when I learned of the idea of erotic slavery. It isn't a science to be learned, though there are lots of skills slaves develop in order to serve more completely.

It begins with some of the core developmental skills that we learn when we are really young: honesty, commitment, determination, and an ability to put someone else before oneself. You must be able to trust and respect, as well, since that allows the master to more completely possess his property.

Some of the more important skills come from what your parents taught you and the skills you learned along the path to becoming an adult. These are the important skills you'll use in service, such as knowing the difference between standing straight and slouching, or how to be respectful and use common courtesy, developing a positive work ethic, the ability to solve problems, honesty and dependability, etc. All of these skills shape an attitude and any master or mistress will benefit greatly if you've learned them well. That's the start of your training process, if you want to be a slave.

I'd also suggest that they are not skills that a master or mistress can easily instill without a great deal of patience and work and time. Old habits die hard, you can't teach an old dog new tricks, you can lead a horse to water, and so on and so forth. Those well used adages are around for a reason. These skills are all foundational; any other training will be undermined without them.

Slavery isn't the magic solution. There is a common desire on the part of slave wannabes to find a master who can shape them and teach them the missing "kindergarten" skills, or "train" them to accomplish things they haven't been capable of achieving on their own. Sometimes, a little structure and guidance can make all of the difference, but in the end, the slave is going to have to find it within himself in order to be successful in these areas. If you can't make some good progress on your own or demonstrate an ability to resolve those issues yourself, it's doubtful that any master or mistress will be able to do it for you.

It has to be the Old Guard way. Many THINK what they want is to be trained the right way, in "Old Guard protocols," without fully understanding that the "Old Guard" were a bunch of individualists, known for doing things in their unique own way. They were suspicious of "rules" and each tended to create what suited him best. Anytime a

‡   See Appendix E.

master opts for what suits him best and fits best into his lifestyle, rather than to try to follow a set of secret rules they think exist, he is following the "Old Guard" tradition. Believe it or not, the "Old Guard" worked from those same "kindergarten" values.

Even *The Real Thing*[§] was written by an individualist who would loathe for you to tell him how to do it.

It's about giving control *rather than someone taking it*. A common complaint from a slave is that he wants more "control" when what he generally means is that he has a fantasy of how things should be and becomes disappointed that the fantasy isn't being fulfilled. There is a difference between serving as your master wants you to serve and serving how you *think* they *should* want you to serve.

There is no universal or standard set of behaviors for slaves, no matter what anyone tries to say. What one master or mistress prefers or thinks is an important protocol might irritate the hell out of another. Far better to wait and be molded in the specifics of your future master than have to unlearn protocols or waste energy on efforts that mean little to someone else. No slave comes to a master or mistress fully trained.

Training is, after all, a relationship-long process.

After Reading Activities

Make a list of activities that you need to do in order to begin, continue, or improve your search for a master. Prioritize the list, as you can't do it all at once. Are there some things that can be acquired easily? Plan to do them first as you make plans and work toward the more difficult or more time-consuming objectives. Write out your plan and give it substance with dates and benchmarks for determining your success.

Are there some things that you might need to know about yourself and/or your new life? List them and then research ways to learn them. You might, for instance, want to get more knowledgeable about Internet searching for a master or in domestic service. In effect, this activity is to help you ascertain what you need to learn in order to become the slave you desire to be.

§   Carney, William, *The Real Thing*, Masquerade Books, Inc., New York, 1995.

7

The Slave's Training

*Being your slave, what should I do but tend
upon the hours and times of your desire?*[*]

As noted earlier, there are two aspects to slavery: The first involves general considerations of the lifestyle itself, such as commitment, attitude, and generally accepted manners. The second set of aspects vary widely from one relationship to another, each being very specialized, tailored by the couple themselves. Whereas the last chapter was devoted to training in general, this one will attempt to be more specific and point out those areas which are often unique from couple to couple.

In that regard, informal training often begins long before the two parties begin serious interviewing and negotiation. It often boils down to the imparting of simple information, meant to guide the process, and then moves on to specifics that illustrate the master-applicant's desires and the slave-candidate's willingness and ability to meet them. As an example, very early on, I "teach" my applicants about my timetable for enthrallment. That gives them an idea of how I am going to proceed.

If we do, indeed, progress, I will request certain forms of behavior, such as calling me "Sir" or responding promptly to e-mails and phone calls. In general, this "training" simply reinforces and explains my expectations concerning "early protocols," as previously discussed.

When a candidate arrives in my living room for a scene, we discuss limits and expectations and I try to answer any lingering doubts or questions. I also share some of the philosophy that I have about the slave's forthcoming experience, some of which will be training. I will tell them, for instance, that they are always free to ask any question,

[*] William Shakespeare in *Sonnet LVII*.

at any time, and that they can expect that I will do the same. Other masters may want to be asked questions only at specific times and under specific circumstances, which is why this instruction is particular, not general in nature.

I also stress that there is much to learn about serving me and that there is no way I can train a slave in every aspect of his service in the short time span of a first meeting. Early training centers on how the slave will address and treat me, as well as the protocols that I will expect him to keep while in my home, such as nudity and not sitting on furniture, except when necessary, such as for eating and using a computer. Other masters have different protocols, such as eating on the floor or wearing a specific uniform.

Understanding the Request

One of the prerequisites for successful training is that the student must understand what is being requested. As stated earlier, I believe it is the responsibility of the trainer to effectively communicate his or her instructions and to monitor the trainee to be sure that the communication was received both correctly and completely.

This is why my methodology differs from those masters who tend to want to keep their slaves "in the dark," why I encourage my slave-applicants and trainees to ask questions, and why I am so quick to seek feedback from them by asking questions such as "How does this feel?" or "What are you thinking?"

When you find yourself in doubt or confusion as to the intent of an instruction, I can only encourage you to find a respectful, yet quick way, to have those questions resolved. A polite request, when necessary, for "permission to speak" is one way to resolve this dilemma. You may also have been given other ways to learn what is needed. In any case, this is hardly a good place for shyness, as not knowing what to do and the proper way to do it will never meet the master's approval.

Though you most certainly may feel differently and there are masters who will act differently as well, it is my opinion that successful long-term relationships are built on the ability of both partners to freely enter into unrestrained dialogue. The master, then, who does not provide opportunities for clarity of communication and improved understanding, may not be the best choice, though I certainly acknowledge that both you and he or she have the right to make choices different from those I make.

Admitting Your Limits

One of the purposes of having scenes before one enters into a full scale relationship is that doing so teaches you a great deal about yourself and your reactions to the various activities that you will encounter in an M/s relationship. As I've written, every relationship is the unique creation of the two (or more) individuals in it. No two are going to be alike and the resulting creation will have to satisfy each participant, at least well enough that they are willing to remain in the relationship.

Master/slave relationships are no different and creating one means that each partner will bring to the relationship his own preferences, desires, and experiences. I can't begin to list the wide variations that are possible, especially when one considers the variables of gender, age, education, vocation, finances, sexual preference, experience, and personality. In fact what all M/s relationships seem to have most in common is the fact that each one is so uniquely the product of the master and the slave.

I know that most people would readily see that the master creates the relationship and most would wonder why I say that both do the creating. Once again, it is the submissive's surrender, his or her willingness to serve, that is a key ingredient in the relationship. Believe me, if such weren't the case, I would have a great many slaves serving me, but the sad (for me) truth is that I was not the master they sought. You, too, will find many masters, most of whom, and perhaps all but one, you will find unsuitable or who you will not suit. It is as simple as that.

The training, too, will reveal the reality of your desire. When fantasy becomes real, it may be much different than your dream life. Often, in fact, training teaches the searcher that what he wants isn't what he thought he wanted, that he really couldn't go where he thought he could.

So, as part of your search, it is important to know your limits: "the point, edge, or line beyond which something cannot or may not proceed." In this case, it is something that you cannot or will not do.

I know that you will find online folks who believe that a slave should have no limits or who say that they have no limits. My response is to remind them that the law of gravity, the money in their checkbook, and the laws of the land each impose limits. Limits are most often thought of as being physical, but they can just as well be psychological, legal, financial, or social.

For the most part, limits pose no problem while developing a relationship; we can and ought to take limits into consideration and most limits are, quite frankly, mutually acceptable. I get a charge, for instance, from slave-applicants who tell me that "scat, blood, and permanent injury" are hard limits. Since I have no intention of doing any of those things anyway, to make them limits doesn't pose a problem. They are, after all, my limits as well.

The problem with limits arises much more often when we discover, sometimes too late, that a limit exists. It is in this situation that we can do no more than to request that the activity stop and then together take stock in what happened. Once again, good relationships are built on good communications and limits are just one more thing that we need to discuss.

On the other hand, you may have some obvious limits that ought to be brought to light sooner, rather than later. If you have, for instance, responsibilities that prohibit you from relocating (such as minor children or elderly parents) then you will have to take them into consideration in your search. If you are unwilling to engage in anal sex, intense pain, or permanent marking, this needs to be mentioned long before you meet to play.

Lastly, if you don't know your limits, be clear about that. Gaining real-time experience will teach you where the boundaries are. We all have them and you not only need them, but can live with them.

Formal Training

Specific training of the slave usually involves the master teaching the slave how he or she likes things done. In that regard it is highly individualized. In most cases, too, it is simply a matter of the master telling the slave to do such and such a specific way and then reinforcing the instruction, as necessary. I am quick to tell new slave-applicants, for example, that there is a great deal to learn about being my slave. The first thing I teach is that the slave is to call me "Sir." From that modest beginning, I will teach him or her thousands of details that I want done for my pleasure.

In some situations, more formal training is necessary. In consultation with the slave, for instance, the master may direct that the slave earn a high school diploma, finish a college degree, or learn a specific skill. I have always wanted (and still do) to find a slave who was a professional masseuse — and am willing to help a slave I own become one!

The slave-applicant needs to evaluate his or her own need for formal training, since in some cases, it might actually be preferable for the slave to finish the training (get the degree) before embarking upon his or her search for a master. In any case, the question is best answered before one enters into a master/slave relationship so both master and slave can be apprised of what kind of formal training (if any) might be needed or desired.

Protocols

As I wrote, though, most training is of the personal kind, unique to the slave's needs and the master's wishes. Perhaps this is nowhere more obvious than in the case of protocols, an often mangled word in our subculture.

Protocol, according to the dictionary, refers to: "The forms of ceremony and etiquette observed by diplomats and heads of state." We kinky folk have taken that word and redefined it to reflect the manners and positions that masters and slaves employ with, between, and among one another. Though there are some general protocols (more appropriately called manners) among Leather folk, for the most part, protocols vary widely; at times, some differ by geographic area. In any case, they are highly dependent upon the will of the dominant.

Once again, I am at a loss to give specifics when it comes to protocols, though I will venture to define them: "The individualized forms of ceremony and etiquette that a slave is required by his or her master to perform." Each and every master will have unique wishes when it comes to being addressed, how a slave will greet him, what to will wear, and how to act.

Warning: This section contains my personal opinion, filled with ranting, and is open to a great deal of contradiction by those who think differently than I do. Therefore, read at your own risk.

A very innocent question once set me off: "Can you advise me on slave positions, SIR? Does one of your books have some information or some website, SIR?" Now, I am sure that the reader who wrote that did so with the best of intentions. He is most likely a serious seeker of slavery, who wants to make sure that he gets it right — even down to the correct way to kneel in front of the master about whom he fantasizes. There's no rant in me about that.

I'm not a search engine, but I do know (since I looked) that a search on Google.com, using "BDSM slave positions," produces some 61,400 web pages that attempt to answer my reader's question. He may want to refer, for instance, to the site that lists and describes the 24 Gorean slave positions: Bara, Belly, Bracelets, Crawl, Gorean Bow, Hair, Heel, Karta, Ko-Lar, Leading Position, Leasha, High Leasha, Nadu, Obediance, Run, She-Sleen, Slaver's Kiss, Slave Lips, Submission, Sula, Sula-Ki, Table, Walk, and Whipping Position.† Of course, since Gorean slaves are female, it might not work for him — but, hey, it's an answer. The problem isn't the answer. The question itself is the problem.

You see, I don't give a damn about 24 positions. My politically incorrect quick answer is "on his back," which I think is a much better answer than High Leasha: "She stands, her back to her Master, with her feet shoulder width apart, her wrists crossed at the small of her back. She holds her head high, turning it to her left, her lips slightly parted

† Visit the World Wide Web at: http://www.geocities.com/Area51/Dimension/6568/posit.htm for more information on these positions.

and lowers her eyes in submission. She awaits his leash."[‡]

Seriously, ranting aside for the moment, the only acceptable position for a slave is that he or she be in the position which, at the moment, pleases the master. That, dear readers, tells you nothing and everything. BDSM, or any of the other terms we use for "what it is that we do," is nothing more than a catch-all euphemism for a great number of highly varied, widely differentiated, and sometimes contradictory human activities. Beyond that, I can write a lot, but say little.

After all, I know several masters very well and am rather well-informed about their slaves' positions. None (except perhaps for the Goreans) require that their slaves do it the same way that another master wishes. Even those who have borrowed from others (and here I include the Goreans), often adapt the posted positions to positions that they, in their own masterful ways, find more pleasing. So, one master requires his slave to walk in front, another (me) at his side, and still a third desires his slave to walk behind. Which position ought my reader learn? The position one's master desires.

The ranting starts when I get the feeling that people think there is one way to do a certain thing correctly. Now, I am all in favor of "my way or the highway" when it comes to my personal relationship with a particular slave, but such a philosophy does not and cannot extend anywhere beyond my own personal relationships. When one begins to think there are "slave positions" that one can learn from a book or a website, then one is missing the point on two counts.

First off, real slave training or any kinky training, for that matter, is an intimate, one-on-one encounter between a person who mentors and one who learns. Yes, it involves reading and searching the Internet and a great number of other activities, but the primary purpose must be the development of a dominant/submissive relationship that is pleasing on a highly individualized level to both the partners. I can teach my reader MY positions, but what he will have learned regarding positions, as such, will be highly individualized and will most likely only work when serving me.

The second point is: The greatest part of what he must learn has little or nothing to do with actual physical positions. Attitude is paramount to what we do. Learn to be trustworthy, mutually respectful, and honorable. Disencumber yourself of those things (people, places, ideas, and habits) that hinder your ability to be all that you want to be. Learn those traits, whatever they might be, that will empower you to attain your full potential.

This isn't just master/slave talk either. Having the right attitude applies to dominants and submissives, to tops, bottoms, and switches,

‡ Ibid.

142

to heterosexuals, gays, and bisexuals equally. Repeat after me: There are no general, across the board, one-answer-fits-all solutions to how one should be kinky. Got that? If not, read it again. Now, I know that sentence is self-contradictory, since it is a generalized and across the board answer. Since I am ranting, please cut me some slack.

There are, of course, generalized and multi-dimensional answers that one can look to for guidance: attend seminars, join a group, discard that which hinders your personal growth, find a mentor, become trustworthy, respectful, and honorable. Yes, you can come to my home for a weekend of training, but the positions I teach you may not work for your next session, scene, or master. On the other hand, the attitude, the decorum, and the presence of mind and heart that you might learn with me will probably suit you well, no matter what the future holds for you.

I am not disparaging technique. The proper application of whip, fist, needle, rope, chain, collar, penis, gag, hood, clamp, catheter, or electrode is always a good idea. Good technique alone, unfortunately, is not enough to create a real Leather person, kinkster, Gorean, lifestyler, or whatever you want to call what you are.

The right attitude is necessary. With the right attitude, one will learn the positions, the techniques, and the protocols. Not only that, but if one has and demonstrates the right attitude, one's ignorance of the "correct position" will matter a great deal less; the perceived attitude is really the single most important defining criterion. Most of what we do is psychological. Our biggest sexual organ is our brain. Without the correct inner disposition, the outer manifestation is nothing more than show — good show maybe, but still show.

That's why we must move past lectures and demonstrations into real person-to-person experiences. That's why cyber BDSM is an empty, pale, and eventually unsatisfying experience. That's why cheaters, braggarts, those who lord, and pretenders are so very disruptive to our groups, our relationships, and our fun.

Going through the motions isn't enough. Your head and your heart have to be in it or it is only empty pretense. Phooey on positions. Have the right attitude and you will automatically find yourself in the right place at the right time. Have the wrong attitude and no amount of correct positioning is going to work. Oh, you can fool some of the people and may even get away with it for awhile, but in the long run, the truth will out and the position will have been for naught.

Slave as Reflection

The real purpose of protocols and training, in general, is the pleasure of the master. It is as simple as that. The way a slave stands, sits, talks, listens, eats, looks, or renders sexual service is important in

143

so far as it gives the master pleasure to have it done in a certain way. Added to that, as if there needs to be another reason, is the plain fact that the slave's appearance, demeanor, and actions reflect directly on the master. If the slave is well-thought of, then the master will be better thought of.

A slave always reflects the master's ability to dominate, control, and train. For better or for worse, the slave greatly influences what others think of the master and there is often no way around this situation. In fact, this "image thing" is a great part of what determines the creation and maintenance of the master/slave relationship. If a master isn't comfortable with the appearance and demeanor of a slave-applicant, he or she is most likely not going to pursue the possibility of enslavement. Put bluntly, we masters all want to find a slave who will not only please us, but who will make us look good, as well.

The Hidden Value of Protocols

There is a side to protocols that is often mentioned, but seldom emphasized. They are necessary actions that help create and maintain the right attitude. We live busy lives with widely different characteristics. We are one kind of person at home, another at work, still a third when visiting our parents, our vanilla friends, or attending a BDSM convention. We wear, to put it mildly, many hats.

Protocols, then, remind us what hat we are wearing. Patrick, for instance, spends his working day focusing on how to increase sales of his company's products. Yes, he is collared and everyone knows that he's "Jack Rinella's slave," but that is not the driving motivation of what he does in that time and place. Upon returning home, he has the requirement of kneeling before me, kissing my feet, and repeating his mantra, each of which reminds both of us that he is my slave and that we will both act accordingly.

In this way, protocols are necessary attitude adjusters and play an important role in maintaining the relationship just where each of the couple wishes it to be.

Demeanor

Several characteristics demonstrate the "correct" slave attitude: one's speech, quietude, an observant and unobtrusive nature, zeal to please, patience, and what I call centeredness. Each of these can be summarized under the rubric of demeanor: "The way in which a person behaves or conducts himself; deportment." Generally, these characteristics, taken together, reflect the slave's humility and recognition of self as submitted and surrendered to the will of his or her master.

This is probably best shown by the way the slave addresses his or her master, such as with the use of the title Sir, Master, my Lord, or my Lady. It extends further than this, though, in that the slave always uses his voice respectfully and does his best to speak in a way that reflects the subservient position.

That neither implies that slaves always agree with their masters nor that they should. Dissent is quite appropriate, as long as it is respectful dissent. Unexpressed dissent holds the real danger that the relationship will be diminished in honesty and openness, and will eventually lead to its ending. Slaves, then, should be heard honestly and openly. Masters ought to encourage their slaves to speak freely and frankly, when the occasion is appropriate.

I have purposely set aside every Sunday night as a time when Patrick can speak in all honesty to me, lest the need to be "slave" somehow destroys the greater need for clear communication between us. Obviously, such conversations need to be more private, lest the ill-informed not understand the dynamic at work. Correction, either of the slave or the master, needs to be a private affair, not a public airing of grievances.

To write that "silence is golden" is to state what ought to be the expected in M/s relationships. Slaves, therefore, are generally expected not to be aggressive in speech, or to speak up unless encouraged to do so, or to interrupt their masters in an intruding and impolite way. Again, this is going to be a more personalized choice on the master's part. I know, for instance, a self-admitted master/slave couple where the slave comes off as quite a loud mouth, but to his credit, his master doesn't seem to mind his speech at all. As long as they are happy, who's to complain?

More generally, and much more widely accepted, is the idea that slaves ought to be more quiet and less noticeable — personality traits not uncommon in many slaves. This is not to deny that several well known slaves are quite good at public speaking and in advising others, making themselves invaluable assets to their owners and to our subculture, as well. This, too, demonstrates that attitude is more important than hard and fast rules when it comes to speech and silence.

Reflecting on the preferred modes for speech and silence, it is generally the custom, expectation, and sometimes even the rule, that slaves need to be unobtrusive — which means "not readily noticeable." They need to be aware of their surroundings and their masters' possible needs, without being bothersome or continually present. When a master has guests, for example, the slave should be aware of the master's will. At times, the master will want to entertain the guest privately, while at other times, the master may invite the slave to participate.

Although informing the slave of his or her wishes is the master's prerogative, slaves often have to either estimate the master's will or simply ask politely. Patrick, for instance, is apt to inquire when I have a dinner guest as to whether he should set the table to include himself or if I prefer to dine privately with my guest. As in this example, asking goes a long way in knowing and maintaining the master's will.

Too often, we equate submissiveness with passiveness. There certainly are times when the slave needs to be passive, but — more often than not — a real zeal to serve, anticipating the master's needs and desires, even staying one step in front of the master, so to speak, can be very helpful. This ability to anticipate the master's will is cultivated only over time, but when the slave achieves such an ability, he or she increases his or her value. On the other hand, one need not always have this sixth sense. As I wrote above, simply asking readily solves the problem of what comes next.

I will return to an earlier statement. Actions speak louder than words. Being proactive, then, can certainly indicate that slave's devotion, his willingness to serve, his surrender to the good of the master. Slaves, remember, have a duty to empower, support, and aid a master's endeavors. Passivity may not be very helpful in this regard, whereas being zealous to please certainly can be.

The actual day to day experience of slavery quickly teaches that much of the slave's time when providing service is spent waiting — thereby making the need for patience more important. Here, we can note a typical double standard: Though the slave is expected to wait upon his or her master's will, slaves should never (even if they do) expect their masters to wait for them. Here is another opportunity for the slave to anticipate his master's next move, being ready to respond to it appropriately.

In all of this, centeredness — the state of being grounded and unflustered — becomes an important characteristic. Keeping one's focus on one's service and one's priorities attuned to those of the master can be a challenging proposition, especially because masters and their slaves quite often have such different personalities. There will, most certainly, be times when serving an overactive, self-centered, and demanding extrovert will drive any selfless introvert crazy. It is then that the slave needs to take a deep breath and remember why he or she has chosen slavery as a lifestyle.

Such times also present a reasonable topic for discussion the next time master and slave have an opportunity to discuss their relationship. Speaking up at the appropriate time always helps a relationship grow and prosper.

Patrick Reflects: Slave Skills

Beyond the growing up values and the other experiences life taught me, the exploring I did in the lifestyle gave me a good foundation of knowledge and skills. The first of what was my "formal slave training" came from the first guy I submitted to for a weekend. I learned more from the second guy, but I learned differently, yet both were correct.

What I learned from them and from others in the lifestyle allowed me to take that and go into scenes with people more confidently, knowing some of what I liked and what I didn't like. When negotiating a scene, it became very easy to agree to do something I hadn't experienced before; my previous experiences taught me to learn to trust and "read" people, to determine who was safe or good to play with and who wasn't. I could feel safe trusting them to do things to me because the other Tops I played with had been worthy of my trust.

So, I learned that a swat to my butt with a crop didn't hurt nearly as much as a swat to my thigh with the same crop, and that a paddle to my butt felt different than the crop did. I could tolerate Japanese clips and then gnat bite clips on my tits, because I'd already experienced clothespins and snakebite suction cups. Alligator clamps looked much less threatening after the gnat bite clips than they did before experiencing the clothespins.

I could also see others in real scenes and gain insight into some of the more advanced stuff, and watch the reactions of others having things done to them that I couldn't yet imagine being done to me. When I did try them out, I sort of knew what to expect.

This means I could learn to trust myself to not bite off more than I could chew, and how to "read" others who approached me to play. Exploring the lifestyle allowed for a certain amount of demystifying of the lifestyle and the people who practiced it. I met others who could explain the difference between a top and a slave, understood that people approached relationships differently, and that our attraction to this lifestyle went more than skin deep. This time of exploring allowed me to better understand why I wanted to be a slave, and the people I explored with encouraged and guided me through the process of looking for a master.

If you think it isn't necessary to involve yourself in the lifestyle before you settle into a long-term relationship with a master, you are being foolish indeed. If you're worried who might see you exploring your desires, take comfort in the realization that those people are exploring THEIR desires, as well. After all, who would better understand and respect your feelings and privacy than they? You aren't going to meet your mother or brother or boss there, and even if you did, all it means is that they are kinky too!

But all of that is the basic stuff we talked about in the last chapter. You've explored and now you are using what you've learned as a basis for learning to be a slave.

When you've found a master, or even as you are auditioning/being auditioned by a prospective master, they will build on what you've learned and show you how to do it their way, the way they like. It doesn't mean the others were wrong, only that your master has his own style.

You see, our community is a collection of individuals — some will say rugged individualists. As such, they are a bunch of individuals who don't hesitate to change, adopt, adapt, create, or ignore "the rules" and techniques, based on their unique tastes and preferences. So, if your exploring taught you how to you stand at attention with your hands at your sides, but someone else tells you that your hands should be clasped behind your neck, they are both correct. If they tie a knot in an odd way or with less attention to detail, it doesn't mean they are wrong; it means they are doing it differently. As long as they understand what it means to be safe, sane and consensual, and you both are practicing risk aware consensual kink (RACK), there isn't a problem and no one is wrong.

When you find your master he or she is going to begin your formal slave training. This means they are going to train you to suck a cock or lick a cunt the way they like it to be done. They are going to teach you how they like towels to be folded; they are going to show you the rituals and protocols they want you to practice.

The first thing Sir taught me was that when my face was in his crotch, my hands should be on his tits. That's how he prefers it and he reinforced that expectation with repetition and ultimately, with punishment, until it became second nature to me. I learned this so well that once he loaned me out to a friend and the friend had me suck his cock. As soon as my mouth closed around his cock, my hands found his tits and started playing with them.

That didn't go over well. He pushed them away. When I was once again fully focused on my task, my hands went right back to his tits without thinking. It took me a moment to realize that Sir's rule wasn't *his* pleasure. He preferred that my hands reach around and massage his ass cheeks while I was sucking!

Sir taught me that the proper way to suck his cock was to take it all the way in and hold it, using my throat muscles and my tongue to massage it, and to learn to breathe around it. My previous master had taught me to do this, but his cock was smaller, and the task was accomplished more easily. So even though I knew the technique, I still had to learn to do it with Sir's more ample cock. It changed the entire technique of learning to breath around the shaft as I did this.

When I moved in, Sir kept his car at a private parking lot near the condo. He taught me that when parking the car, it had to be parked front end in. It seemed to me it was more logical to park it nose out, as it was easier to back into the space than to back out of it. The first time I did that, he had to explain that if it wasn't parked front first, then when security came to check the parking lot, if they couldn't see the parking sticker in the window, they would tow the car away. That was one slave skill I learned quickly!

But each to his or her own. They all were correct, they just had their own way of wanting things. Learning the specifics of what your specific master wants is what slave training is all about. When you weren't a slave, you learned certain skills. When you become a slave, you have to learn how to adapt those skills to your specific master's preferences. You'll learn additional skills as well — things you might not have had a clue about before, but when they are learned well, it means you learned to do them in the manner your master wants them done.

This is why it is important to explore the lifestyle. You will learn skills that your master or mistress can refine and adapt to his or her needs and desires. And much of what you learn in your exploring will not only be acceptable as is to your new master, but it will also allow you to be more confident in yourself as you enter into this relationship because it won't be all a mystery.

After Reading Activities

Search the Internet for an SM-related questionnaire or use the one in Appendix B to make a list of the various fetish and other aspects of a M/s relationship that may present limits to you (e.g., fisting, scat, or relocation to a different state or country). Reflect on your limits. Are there some that you might overcome? Are there some that make your slave search more difficult or unreasonable? If so, how might you mitigate the restrictions these limits place on your success?

If you feel the need for some type of formal training, investigate it more fully. Is it compatible with your search for a master? Is it something to include in your slave bio? Ought you set aside your search for a master until your formal education is complete?

Use your journal to describe how you perceive your demeanor. Is it appropriate to your ability to become a master's slave? How can you communicate this to a prospective master? Does it influence the type of master you will need to find? If so, how?

8

The Role of Punishment

*He who spares the rod hates his son, but he
who loves him is diligent to discipline him.*[*]

. The process of selecting a partner requires a great deal of communication, though that is neither assurance that you will succeed in either selecting nor in communicating. For that reason, I have learned to do a lot of writing and talking about the relationship with my prospect before I make any commitment to enter into a relationship for any time longer than a weekend. It's a process of getting to know you, getting to know all about you.

In one case, since it was to be a long distance relationship, I was a bit more challenged than usual when it came to some of its aspects, particularly punishment. When D/s partners live with one another, communication (for good or bad) can happen quickly and without a great deal of effort or planning. Likewise, transgressions are more easily noted and corrective measures taken. When miles separate them there are a whole set of issues that change that dynamic. I can hardly spank someone over the phone.

There is more to it than that, of course. Living together gives me the opportunity to encourage and support, and to give ready explanation of why I want such a thing in such a way. Distance, on the other hand, means that many of the benefits that should be available to my slave, will have to be delayed until we can be together again. This means it is more difficult for him to be mindful of my will and to remain in a mind space appropriate to service and submission.

Before I go on about punishment, though, let me set a few guidelines. First, rules must be stated clearly, understood, and mutually agreed

---

[*] *Old Testament*, Proverbs, chapter 13, verse 24, *Revised Standard Version*.

upon. They ought to have purpose and value. We are not making rules to trick someone into being punished. We masters have the right, given to us by our slaves, to do what we want. Without that right, I am not in control and therefore, cannot make rules. Likewise, I don't need a transgression as an excuse to do what I wish to do. I am a sadist, for instance, and can beat him whenever I like, with no need to wait for some misbehavior to justify my sadism.

I make rules for my pleasure. That is, I make rules so that my slaves behave in a way that pleases me. They are very personal and have more to do with my desires and how I want to live than for any other reason. For instance, I find enjoyment in seeing a slave naked or collared. It pleases me to know he is abstaining from sexual gratification or that he is exercising at a gym to please me.

Rules are also meant to help a slave maintain a proper attitude of submission. They act as fences to keep him in his proper mental space. So, for instance, Patrick has a rule about kissing my feet to greet me. Doing so reminds both of us as to why he is with me. Another rule is that he addresses me as "Sir" at all times, which does the same thing. It is a matter of being in the correct mental state, something that benefits everyone, no matter what their relationship or state. Who, after all, wants to have a bad attitude or be around someone who has one?

Having agreed upon the rules and having submitted to them, there needs be a consequence for disobedience. It must be a negative consequence as well, lest the disobedience be encouraged. You see, if I have authority it must be exercised or it is pointless. Authority has limits too; so punishments should fit the crime so to speak and be non-injurious to body, emotions, or relationship.

Punishment is meant to be cathartic — that is it clears the air and gives finality to the transgression. Once punished, forever gone, is the proper way to do it. It is meant to be corrective as well, in that it fosters behavior modification. It is a matter of reinforcing correct actions and giving negative reinforcement to unwanted ones. For that reason, punishment is reactive, after the fact.

Sometimes it's easier to discuss punishment by saying what it is not. For instance, anger has no place in punishment. I try my best (and most often succeed) to never punish in anger, as it is then not a force for correction, but one for propagating more anger. So, it's obvious that one does not punish in anger, but that it is necessary, when the situation angers, that the anger be first dispelled, then the punishment be administered.

Punishment is often confused with discipline and with sadomasochistic activity. It is neither. A discipline is a regimen imposed on oneself or another to produce a desired effect. So, I discipline myself not to eat dessert so that I will lose weight. On the other hand, if I were to disobey a rule, I might be punished by having my dessert withheld for a week. See the difference? The actions look alike, but one is *a priori*, in order to have a future effect, while the other is reactive in order to dissuade one from acting that way again in the future.

In our subculture, we often use the word discipline as another term for sadomasochistic activity. SM, for us, is meant to be pleasurable erotic behavior. We do it because it arouses us and thereby, creates delightful physical and emotional states. Whipping, flogging, and spanking are often called "discipline," though that use of the word doesn't conform to the dictionary. Vocabulary aside, SM should always be clearly differentiated from punishment. One is for fun, the other for correction. Confusing or obscuring the purpose of either will corrupt and degenerate both.

I don't think that empty threats are appropriate either. I know what I want and I hope I am properly communicating that to my slave. I don't think it is threatening to say that such-and-such an activity will displease me and in order to discourage it, I will punish its appearance. As master, that is my right. For the slave, then, it is a take it or leave it proposition. I suppose there is only a slight difference between warning and threatening, but you get my point. Threatening destroys security. Slaves must be secure in their place, their role, and their relationship. Punishment is meant to be corrective and supportive, not destructive.

If warnings are given and not heeded, and then the master fails to follow through on his word, he greatly endangers his credibility, erodes the slave's trust in him, and casts serious doubt on his credibility. For these very serious reasons, masters need to take care that their rules are reasonable, viable, and clearly communicated, and that the punishments are warranted by the transgression.

Another point about rules is that the master leads by example, as well as by dictum. That means that the master is required to live up to his rules, such as by being protective and supportive, and has to remember the rules he has given to his slave. This is the best reason for KISS (keep it simple, stupid), as there are few things that will make a master's rules look foolish than the fact that the master doesn't know what they are. If they are not important enough for the master to remember, they certainly aren't important enough for enforcement. If they aren't being implemented, they ought to be discarded.

In reality, there is very little punishment in a typical master/slave relationship. I certainly will grant that those just entering the life of slavery have much to learn and punishment, when administered judiciously, can expedite their education. On the other hand, experience shows that slaves learn quickly and want to please, thereby usually making punishment that much less necessary.

I can honestly say that punishment is never a pleasure. It is a responsibility and represents a failure on the part of both the master and the slave. It does not please me to have a slave disobey. I don't need disobedience to enjoy beating him, or to do anything else I want to do. For that reason, it is important that rules be clearly communicated and understood. I am firm in my practice of warning before I punish. I am careful to give warning with words like "That was against my rule and if you do it again, I will punish you." Punishment is simply a form of training and it is the master's responsibility to train responsibly.

A Contrary Opinion

You've noticed, I'm sure, that a good deal of what is in this book is my opinion. Yes, it is based on experience, but the wide variety of modalities in living the M/s relationship makes it nearly impossible to standardize many of the particular ways masters and slaves fashion their partnerships. Punishment offers just such a difficulty.

The idea of punishing is a difficult and often controversial concept. At times, I have had serious reservations about the efficacy of corporal punishment. More often, though, I have seen it as useful and productive. The best example I have of this occurred early in my own submission to Master Lynn. At the time, my body had the tendency to ejaculate rather easily and while talking with him on the phone one evening, I had an orgasm without his consent. It earned me ten whacks with a shaving strop the next time I was at his home. Some week or so later, while playing with my new master, I came a second time without permission. It was back to the cellar and the strop once more. The combined punishments made it easier for me to contain my jism and the spontaneous orgasms stopped. It was then that I realized that punishment works.

Other masters consider corporal punishment unnecessary or even detrimental to the relationship and therefore, rely on psychological punishment, reasoning, or (a very few) ignoring the transgression altogether. Some believe that only positive reinforcement is effective. One reader responded to a column I wrote about punishment with the suggestion that I read the book, *Don't Shoot the Dog*, which recommends that only positive reinforcement is effective. It is interesting that the author notes that punishment is a form of domination. That makes me think it is appropriate in the master/slave relationship, something that she doesn't venture to write about.

Punishing is also reinforcing for the punisher because it demonstrates and helps to maintain dominance. Until the day when a boy is big enough to hit his brutal father back, the father feels dominant and is, in truth, the dominant one. This in fact may be the main motivation behind our human tendency to punish: establishing and maintaining dominance. The punisher may be primarily interested not in behavior, but in being proved to be of higher status.[†]

The general consensus arrived at in my interviews, though, is that punishment of some kind is effective. This opinion, surprisingly enough, is held not only by dominants, but by many slaves as well. Administered properly, punishment is generally thought of as being highly cathartic, bringing atonement[‡], satisfaction, and closure to actions that admittedly have disrupted the relationship.

Proper Punishment

What then are the guidelines one ought to follow if one has decided that punishment is a useful tool in the training and correction of a slave? First of all, as mentioned above, punishment should never be administered in anger. That's not to say that a slave's transgression won't anger the master as it most certainly can do so. What it means is that the master needs to take care that if there is anger, it is dealt with within him or herself so that the punishment arises out of a sense of correction, instruction, or atonement and not of anger. I usually approach my own anger at my slave by admitting that I am angry and informing him that whatever it is that made me angry will have to be discussed and dealt with once my anger has subsided.

Just as importantly, I never punish when the infraction was caused by a lack of information. Only rules that are well known to the slave are rules that can be "broken" by the slave. It is, therefore, necessary that the master fully communicate any wishes or prohibitions and be certain that the submissive understands their importance and that their omission or violation will bring some kind of punishment.

For that reason, new trainees are seldom punished at the first infraction. Instead, I am in the habit of reminding them of the rule that they have broken and giving them a warning that future violations will incur a punishment. First time offenders may, in fact, receive nothing more than a symbolic or greatly decreased punishment. Repeated infractions, however, warrant direct and full correction.

In my home, this means ten whacks on the bare ass with a very painful clothes brush, used almost exclusively for punishment. The whack are administered quickly and without warm-up. They are neither sadistic nor pleasurable. The brush has had its bristles pulled out, leaving the wood

---

† Pryor, Karen, *Don't Shoot the Dog! The New Art of Teaching and Training*, Revised Edition, Bantam Books, New York, 1999, ISBN 0-553-38039-7

‡ Atonement means "Amends or reparation made for an injury or wrong; expiation." To atone, then, means to reconcile or harmonize, to conciliate, appease.

handle riddled with small holes that increase its pain. Other masters have other means of punishing, such as deprivation, assigning tasks that are disagreeable to the slave, isolation, the writing of an essay, or writing "I will not disobey this rule" a thousand times by hand.

If the rule is one that the slave repeatedly violates, one needs to enter into a serious dialogue with the slave as to why such violations continue to occur. Punishment without some kind of dialogue that leads to increased understanding and more appropriate behavior is rather useless punishment.

I once had a slave move in under less than ideal circumstances, as his roommate was demanding that he move out and the interview process itself was rushed. Before accepting my collar, I gave him my expectations, which included (among others) two rules: the first was that he was not to smoke cigarettes, and the second was that he was to abstain from the use of alcohol. As an aside, this second rule applied only to him, as I found, during our negotiations process, that he had a tendency to drink until he was drunk. I suspected alcoholism, but could not confirm it. As I said, the negotiation process was unfortunately rushed.

In any case, for better or for worse, the candidate moved in. Things actually went quite well for the first few months and I was feeling very hopeful about our relationship. One Tuesday night while we were having sex, I happened to kiss my slave, and to my surprise tasted tobacco on his breath. I told him so and said that we would deal with it later, at a more appropriate time. The next evening, I told him that I was quite upset with what to me seemed like a serious betrayal.

His response was to advise me to beat the hell out of him and get it over with. I was, in fact, still too angry to do so. I also felt that the smoking was indicative of a deeper problem. This was confirmed the next day when my slave, Patrick, confided in me that one of the bottles of whiskey, which was rarely used, had been practically drained of its contents. Someone was drinking in secret.

Herein, then, was a serious dilemma. The breaking of two rules was secondary to the violation of our contract. This slave was being secretive and deceptive. There was, I thought, no amount of pounding on his butt that would adequately confront this problem. The slave then began to try to negotiate with me through e-mail, even though we were living in the same house. I delayed having a conversation with him about the matter until Friday night.

I then told him how I felt and why, and suggested that the problem was that he didn't know me well enough and therefore, was unable to be open and honest with me about his problems and difficulties. I suggested that I remove his collar and that he live with us for a month to get to know me as a person before he once again submitted himself to me as a slave.

This suggestion provoked a great deal of anger on his part. He warned me that if I took the collar off that would be the end of our relationship and that he would just go out that night, get drunk, and have a hell of a good time. He then went on to accuse me of lying to him about my ability to support him financially in order to induce him to become my slave. Needless to say, the collar came off immediately. The man was never actually punished, as he did in fact, go out that night, got drunk, and was found the next morning asleep on the living room floor with a very unwelcome trick.

If, in fact, I had tried to punish him while angry, we would obviously have had quite a shouting match. Beyond that, too, interrupting a sexual encounter is no way to administer punishment. There needs to be a clear delineation between punishment and erotic play. Note, too, that effective punishment must first determine the reason for the transgression, show that it was intentional, and be directly related to the cause of the transgression. If I had merely punished him for smoking, then none of the real issues (drinking or his anger at my financial situation) would have been addressed.

Punishment needs to be a private affair as well, though there are some masters who enjoy humiliation as a punishment. I, too, enjoy humiliating my slaves, but that is in the context of erotic play, not in developing a strong, lasting, and mutually pleasing relationship.

Though there are often reasons to delay punishment, the delay needs to be reasonable and of rather short duration, lest the details of the infraction be forgotten over time. Be careful, too, that there not be a great delay, since punishment brings closure, which might be actually needed by both of you. Likewise, needlessly delaying punishment sends a signal that the infraction didn't matter much or that the master is not concerned with the quality of the slave's obedience. For that reason, masters need be very much concerned that rules be not overly burdensome, unrealistic, or of no real value. Especially note that an unenforceable rule, or one that the slave cannot obey, is harmful to the master/slave relationship and ought to be avoided.

As I began this chapter, long distance or part-time relationships especially call for obedience to reasonable and livable rules. There is no profit in creating rules solely that the slave will be forced to break them. Masters need no reason to enjoy their slaves sadistically if they wish. Sadism, though, has no part in punishment and the two must be carefully distinguished from one another. Masters who set their slaves up for failure are doing nothing to foster a healthy relationship.

Needless to say, punishment must not be injurious to the health of the body, the mind, or the relationship. We are looking here for correction, for improvement in the overall quality of the master/slave relationship, and anything that undermines the relationship needs to be strictly avoided.

Deprivation

It is very probable here that I am in the minority when it comes to the use of deprivation as punishment, simply because I believe that if I deprive my slave, I may, in fact, be depriving myself and I am too selfish to do so. I suppose I could order my slave to refrain from using the Internet, make him eat dog food from the floor, or make him stay in his room every night for a week. It's my feeling (and this may be a minority opinion) that such actions would turn out to be counter-productive, instilling a sense of anger, not obedience, in my slave.

On the other hand, if I had several slaves (and yes, I'm looking), I could more easily deprive one slave if I had others on hand to take up the slack. I have long fantasized, for instance, that refusing to allow my slave to suck my dick would be an excellent punishment. Unfortunately, with only one slave mouth in the house, I'm not willing to deprive myself, as well. I'll leave that to more stoic masters.

Patrick Reflects: When it REALLY Hurts!

Punishment is, I think, considered by many non-D/s types to be a silly concept in our little corner of the lifestyle. Most simply see punishment as an exterior part of our play, a physical thing, merely an excuse to segue into a specific scene. Many Tops misunderstand it as a reason to move into more severe or extreme play, or even as an opportunity to briefly step over a limit: "I told you if you didn't repeat it correctly you would be severely punished."

In a short-term, scene-oriented relationship, punishment is often part of the play and then it's all about giving pain that the slave wraps their head around to enjoy. In an ongoing master/slave relationship punishment becomes a more serious affair. Master/slave relationships are built upon a foundation of rules and trust and when a trust is betrayed or a rule broken it can often be handled by the master dispensing corrective punishment. It is less a physical punishment and more of a psychological/emotional issue.

The following is an excerpt from the journal I kept during the first two years of my slavery and I hope it shows the more emotional nature of punishment in a M/s relationship. Though I don't recall the specific disobedience, I apparently didn't have something done when I was supposed to be done. Usually, in a case like this, Sir would have given me more than one deadline, so the issue was less one of lack of time and more one of not taking the time to complete something.

4th, Tuesday, PM — *My Master is home. All weekend long I tried not to miss him, tried to pretend he was at Michael's because I'm used to that. But tonight it feels very good to have him back home. He'll be at Michael's tomorrow night but that's no problem. It was generous of Michael to give us the time tonight together.*

When I got home and realized Michael wasn't here I thought, "Oh, no." All day long I had kept thinking that I had to find time to get those receipts sorted and ready so I could zip through and get them entered. I was sure they wouldn't get home until later and that I could go upstairs first thing and take care of it. When Sir came home alone I really didn't know how to feel, hoping he wouldn't bring up the subject but I knew I wouldn't get through the night without his asking. The whole time I was fixing dinner I felt guilty and stupid. I couldn't fully enjoy having him home with the suspense of that hanging over me. I almost brought the subject up myself but he mentioned about having to deal with plants on the deck and so I waited. When he did bring the subject up I was so relieved; finally it was out in the open and I could quit fretting about it. I knew it wouldn't please him but at least it was no longer a fear.

A friend of Sir's stopped over for a bit and while he was here I went in and got down the brush. I wanted it over with so the issue could be laid to rest. He said that after his master punishes him he still reminds him of past mistakes and I don't think I could deal with that happening very often. Sir works from a clean slate and it makes it much more enjoyable to serve him, as I always know where I stand with him.

And then, later in the bedroom when I thought he might not punish me, I didn't know what to think. I really didn't want to be beaten by the brush but I wanted to be able to enjoy the rest of the evening and I knew I couldn't do that If he didn't punish me. When he laid back in bed I thought, "Good, he is not going to use it." Then he sat back up had me lay over his lap, and I thought "Good, he is going to use it." When he began talking I thought maybe he would just punish me verbally, letting me know that he was being patient but was disappointed. As he rubbed my ass with his hands, though, I knew I was going to get it. And I also know it was the best thing. Then I could get wholeheartedly into his use of me.

Punishment means I have failed to do my part of what is expected of me and have created a break in the relationship. By punishing me, Sir is allowing me the opportunity to mend that break and move the relationship forward. It cleans the slate and ends the issue. Punishment is a last resort kind of thing, as usually problems or issues are approached in positive ways that create a learning experience. But when failure does occur, it's a good way of allowing the emotions of the moment to find rest and letting the relationship continue on with a positive spirit.

After Reading Activities

What do you think of punishment? Were you punished as a child? There are two questions for your journal or to ask at the next BDSM discussion group you attend.

Do some research at the library or on the Internet to learn about punishment. Why might it be helpful and why not? How will you discuss this with your future master?

9

The Small and Not-So-Small Stuff

If you're not courageous enough to make yourself take the risks, then I suggest that you go out and insert yourself into programs designed to help you find your own bravery within yourself.[*]

Fear

It's important to speak about the first stumbling block encountered in developing a committed M/s relationship: our fear of failure. Fearing to fail is hardly the exclusive characteristic of one group or personality trait, but I have concluded that it presents a serious hesitation, to say the least, to many aspiring slaves. Over and over again while interviewing potential slaves, I run into questions that indicate that the applicant has misgivings about his or her ability to succeed.

This fear applies to more than just slave-applicants, of course. Newbies, top or bottom, feel the same insecurity, as if they think that we expect neophytes in our midst to come with all the requisite experience and confidence needed to act like the "oldest guard" among us. That expectation is nonsense, but holds sway, nonetheless.

I was reminded of that fact one Friday, when a man I'll call Charles, came to my house. We had a passing acquaintance with one another, though that date was prompted by an e-mail which he sent me, asking if I would trade a computer education for his serving me in any way I might like. Such an opportunity is always worth investigating, so I asked him over to talk and have dinner.

No failure here. His e-mail was cautious and even belittled his proposal

---

[*]   A grateful slave with Guy Baldwin, M.S., *SlaveCraft, Roadmaps for Erotic Servitude*, Daedalus Publishing Company, Los Angeles, CA, 2002.

161

a bit, but I received it well. Even at this stage of the communication, we fear to fail. Most often, we expect that the failure will be in the form of rejection, which no one, and I mean no one, wants to happen. This fear is so strong that it often paralyzes us so that the initial question isn't even asked. OK, folks, nothing ventured, nothing gained. If you don't take that initial risk, you'll never get the answer you want.

But Charles got a "yes," and so came over to talk. Since I, too, fear failure, I structure my first meetings with little or no expectations. All I plan to do is meet and find out enough about the person to ascertain whether we should proceed. With that kind of agenda, I can't fail, since deciding not to proceed is an acceptable outcome.

Happily for me, Charles presented a very attractive offer. His body was well-muscled and smooth, the body-builder type over which every (well almost every) person drools. He was obviously intelligent and industrious. The smile on his face and in his eyes was incredibly inviting. I appreciated his SM experience, his roguish willingness, and his obvious high sex drive. This was a keeper.

I quickly increased my expectations and invited him to stay for dinner, but duties at home prevented him from staying. That fear of failure came upon me, though not too seriously, as I hoped that he would come back soon. So, the next day I hopped on the phone and invited him to come to dinner on Friday night at 6 P.M. He graciously assented. Nonetheless, when the phone rang at 5:55 and I heard Charles' voice, I thought he was calling to cancel. Fear is such a devious emotion, rearing its ugly head whenever it pleases. There was no need for it here, as Charles was only calling to say that he was running late.

Dinner went well and we adjourned to the deck to talk, since I felt foolish about conducting him directly from dessert to the bedroom. The deck provided a safe space to transit into sex. We sat under the stars for a while and got to know a bit more about one another. Knowledge is power, and knowing your partner is the single most important way to keep your relationship alive and growing. When we cease to know each other, problems arise, especially when one of the partners changes without the other catching on.

As important as it is for the top to know the bottom, the same can be said for the bottom. There is no need to fear, but there is the need to understand one another, to read the nuances of voice and body language, to know each other's dreams and passions, as well as fears and doubts. That's why rushing into a relationship isn't a very good idea. Take time to know one another, to get past the fears that hold you back, and your partnership will be richer and deeper for having done so.

I might note that the fears here may not seem to be very substantial, but they are, nonetheless real. Too often, it is the small stuff that we sweat.

Eventually lust won out and I invited Charles to come downstairs into my bedroom. Despite my fears and perhaps because of his, he was a willing and delightful partner. I won't go into the sexy details, but at every turn of a muscle, every roll on the bed, and every slap, restraint, kiss, and feel, he responded with gusto, eventually bringing me to sexual ecstasy.

Now, the problem with having sex with someone for the first time is that we don't really know what the other expects or how they will react. My slave, Patrick, has long known that when I shoot, I practically become comatose, enjoying in quiet the sensations that accompany my orgasm, until I drift off into sleep. Charles, on the other hand, since this was the first time we had sex, had no such information. He had no way to know what to do when I became so quiet. It's now that fear takes over once more and he projects that something is wrong. Of course, it isn't. But fear knows no rationality and feeds upon projection of self into the situation. It grows with uncertainty, self-doubt, and a self-image expecting to fail.

As he left for the night, I knew that it had gone really well and that I wanted to pursue this guy for all I'm worth; so, I made a mental note to call him the next day. I suspected, too, that my crashing on him might have left him confused, that fear of having failed would rear its ugly head.

When we talked the next evening, he expressed his concern as to whether or not I had been pleased. Of course I was. I even joked that the next time we had sex, I would have a set of cards numbered one to ten under the bed so that when we were done, I would have an easy way to communicate a job well done. Communication, you see, is the best antidote to fear. If trust is the foundation of our relationships, then knowledge is the material with which it's built. Discussing our fears with one another and understanding why we feel a certain way paves the way to a real freedom of acting and relating without fear.

This is a two-way street, as well. Partners, whether prospective, long-term, or somewhere in between, need to share their fears and help one another to overcome them. For that reason, I often tell slave-applicants that it's the master's responsibility to help them succeed. Tops who purposefully set their bottoms up for failure "so that they can be punished," and bottoms who fail on purpose for the same reason, are adversely affecting their relationships.

Fear is not an easily dispelled feeling and there is probably no one way, and certainly no best way, to deal with it. There are, though, several things that you can do to overcome it:

163

- Acknowledge it.
- Understand it.
- Get the facts.
- Weigh the risks
- Take appropriate action.

Denial never helps, and fears — even of the most imagined sorts — are real in their effect. What you fear is real to you, even if it has absolutely no reality, except in your imagination. Therefore, the first step in dealing with fear is to acknowledge that it exists. Admit it to yourself. Write about it in a journal. Share your feelings with someone you can trust, especially someone who has some kind of experience with what you fear. There is nothing as healthy as light to dispel shadow. Some ten years, ago my slave, Patrick's, big fear, for instance, was that he didn't think anyone would understand his desire for slavery, that others would make fun of it, belittling his willingness to take a "sex game" so seriously. That fear hindered his ability to get his life ready for slavery. Recognizing that there were those who did appreciate his desire helped him to overcome his fear.

Having allowed that there is fear, you can now look at it with an eye to understanding it. What exactly do you fear? Are your fears financial? Health-related? Do you fear rejection? Failure? Ridicule? Injury? Loss of friends, family, or employment? Just as importantly, why do you fear what you fear? Are there experiences in your past that reinforce your fear? Are there similar traits in your family? What "tapes" are playing in your subconscious? What rules were you taught that make what you fear seem more real to you? Put into context, many people haven't taken a therapeutic look at themselves to understand, and thereby deal with, the tapes and the rules left over from their childhood and adolescence. Reading and applying this book might well be the first step, though I wholeheartedly suggest professional counseling (if necessary) and books on self-help.

Many fears are based upon some kind of misconception. Of course, there are some things that ought to be feared, such as a frayed wire or a tornado, but most are based on a lack of knowledge about the actual possibility of danger. For that reason, getting the facts from an expert is an important step. Is your fear health-related? Talk to a competent doctor. Is it scene-related? Find an experienced player.

What kind of misinformation do you have that might be making your fear more formidable? What myths do you harbor that help paint a paranoid picture? Though your fears may be founded in some kind of reality, they are most probably made more intense by the various fictions that you believe. The transformation from a single person to that of master or slave will necessitate a change in at least some of your beliefs. What are the beliefs that hold you back, that whisper failure and defeat to your inner hearing?

Examples of misinformation are rampant. Many, for instance, believe that becoming a slave means that they must sever all ties with their biological families. Aspiring masters might believe that they have to appear stoic, that any expression of emotion is inappropriate and a sign of weakness. We might, for instance, have the habit of taking rejection personally, when in fact "no" may have nothing at all to do with us.

Only after we have the facts can we weigh the risks. I admit that we're never going to have all the facts and that information is elusive and seldom complete. Nevertheless, we can often get enough information to make an educated guess about outcomes, to weigh the pros and cons to see what is really the most reasonable, and the safest, path of action. We are never (well hardly ever) going to eliminate all doubt and fear, but we can understand the risks: "the possibility of suffering harm or loss; danger." Since risk indicates possibility, we can then rank it as to its probability. In all likelihood, that which we fear will not come upon us. It may be possible, but its occurrence is highly unlikely. Only facts will help you estimate the danger.

Safer Sex†

One of the areas where fear most often raises its ugly specter is that of sexually transmitted disease. Though safer sex has justifiably become a hallmark of the fight against the spread of HIV and AIDS, there are a host of other STDs that one needs to guard against. In fact, many STDs are more prominent and more easily transmitted than HIV.

The best antidote to fear about disease is to become informed about safer sex guidelines and to practice them faithfully.

I'm not going to go into all the details of safer sex, but I will emphasize the need for it. Simply put, play with every partner as if the person were infected. Never share toys that aren't sterilized between uses, never do anything that transfers bodily fluids‡ between individuals, and don't endanger your health with immune-suppressive activity, such as drunkenness and drug abuse.

What, then, are slaves and masters to do? My Expectations and Regulations spell it out this way: "Once the slave is the Master's property, the Master will be responsible to keep him as healthy as possible. The

† This section is a condensation of a similar essay in my book, The Compleat Slave.

‡ This prohibition reflects a conservative view concerning HIV transmission. Once again, I am not a health professional and can only strongly advise you to consult one for the best and safest advice.

Master will want to keep his property at full value and so will not command or treat the slave in a way that jeopardizes or diminishes his value. A healthy slave is a valuable one."

Not everyone looks at it this way, of course. We frequently see ads that seek "HIV negative" slaves or hear talk about using condoms only "until your slavery is permanent." In both cases, there is the as yet unspoken, but all too obvious, idea that there are conditions within which safer sex practices can be ignored. That kind of thinking only leads to eventual tragedy.

I will exempt married, heterosexual couples, in a monogamous relationship. Other than that, there is no reason to disregard illness-preventing guidelines. If you are unsure of what that means, I strongly encourage you to talk to your physician or county health professional to become informed.

It's a matter of common sense and "risk management." I don't think we can eliminate all risk. The only completely safe sex is no sex, just as the only completely safe kind of travel is to stay home. If you do that, then you can't blame your accidents on traveling. They will happen. On this planet death is the only way out. That doesn't mean, though, that we ought to be courting death or doing things that make it more likely to occur.

Care doesn't mean abstinence. In fact, there are endless erotic possibilities in SM. The vast majority of leather activity is safe, and even the most kinky practices can be made safer with a bit of forethought. The overriding considerations are cleanliness and the use of barriers against the transmission of disease. Keeping ropes, slings, whips, gags, dildos, and the like, clean, is a perfect job for any slave. There's nothing expensive about soap and water. Rinsing insertable toys in bleach (diluted in water in a ration of one to ten) is highly recommended, as well.

Leather toys may not stand up to washing like a butt plug would, but there are ways to disinfect them, as well. See "Leather And Latex Care: How To Keep Your Leather And Latex Looking Great."[§]

Returning to the idea that "A healthy slave is a valuable one," brings us to considering the possibility of conflict in the master/slave scenario. What happens if a Master wants to fuck his slave without a rubber or if the slave wants it to happen? There are those, I'm sure, who will say that the Master has a right to fuck in any way he desires. I understand the sentiment. Rubbers diminish the intensity of the action. They can be a distraction from the heat of the moment. Some men can't stay erect when they put a rubber on. Despite those possibilities, condoms prevent

§   Thibault, Kelly, *Leather And Latex Care: How To Keep Your Leather And Latex Looking Great*, ISBN 1-881943-00-3, Daedalus Publishing Co., Los Angeles, 1996.

infection and thereby, save lives.

It's a matter of getting used to them. Try different brands, sizes, and kinds. For a long time, I relied on the free condoms distributed at the bars. They work well and it was easy to grab a handful as I was going home. I had problems with them, though, in as much as very often they were too tight, so tight, in fact, that more often than not, when I had an orgasm in one, it would be painful. I found ways to avoid that. For one, I would rip off the condom and shoot my load elsewhere and safely. Interestingly, many bottoms enjoyed the sight of my jism squirting onto their chests. Later, I tried a larger size of condom and found they delivered greater pleasure, eliminating the disagreeable tightness. It's a matter of trial and error. Often, too, it's a matter of just getting used to them. By and large it all goes back to being responsible.

There are a great many aspects to Leather sex: pleasure, authority, sadomasochism, love, dominance and submission. You get the idea. None of them removes the need to be responsible. Responsibility is a major attribute between SM players. Without it, the master/slave relationship, or any relationship for that matter, quickly deteriorates and ends. It's a two-way street, too.

The Master is such because he accepts responsibility as part of his role. The slave accepts that his Master is responsible, though he or she still retains self-responsibility, as well, even if only to ensure that the Master's property remains healthy and of great value. As Master, I pass some of my responsibility on to my slave. He is required, for instance, to clean the toys, to buy the condoms, and to put them on me. In the heat of passion, a responsible Master might have to remind his or her slave to get a rubber. It's all part of a healthy relationship and keeping it that way.

The Next Problem

Fear is often accompanied and, in fact, may be caused by doubt. Like fear, doubt can be helpful as a sign not to proceed and there are very real circumstances in which one should not proceed. Doubt, too, has a cure. Dispelling doubt is important because unless we do so, our ability to trust, the basis of any healthy relationship and the foundation of all our kinky play, will be severely hampered. Though we may enter into a relationship, a fetish, or a scene with some amount of doubt, chances are that unless we resolve our doubts they will plague us incessantly and eventually destroy that which we wish to create.

Even my dictionary demonstrates the close relationship between doubt and trust, when it defines the verb form of doubt as: "To be undecided or skeptical about; to tend to disbelieve; distrust." The noun form does the same: "A lack of conviction or certainty; A lack of trust;

[and] A point about which one is uncertain or skeptical."

Doubt will never be fully eliminated from our human situation, as certainty, "a clearly established fact" is rarely possible, especially when it involves human feelings, relationships, and outcomes. What we can attain is a high degree of confidence in the certainty of a given answer. It is this probability of correctness that we must use as the basis for our decision-making, lest we find ourselves incapable of action.

I am, therefore, saying that we don't need to eliminate all doubt. Doing so isn't possible, any more than it is possible to eliminate all fear. What is important is that we find ways to mitigate our doubts so that we have a high probability of being correct, a probability of success that is higher than that of failure.

The process for eliminating doubt centers around our confidence in the validity of what is true in a given situation. Notice that the dictionary calls the focus of our doubt "a point about which one is uncertain or skeptical." Resolution of doubt, then, hinges on recognizing this "point," that instance of fact which presents uncertainty to us. I write this because by definition doubt is based on a specific area of information. This being so, the process of dealing with doubt begins with being able to state the "fact" whose certainty is in question. Resolving doubt is much like resolving fear. We must first be able to acknowledge it, to understand what it is we are doubting. Are we doubting ourselves in this situation or is it someone or something external to us that is causing us to doubt?

My experience is that most doubt is internal. The person giving us the information and, therefore, whom we are doubting is ourselves. This kind of doubt, obviously, is much more difficult to resolve, since it is an inner conflict. If we are doubting an external fact, others can more easily confirm the trustworthiness of the fact, thereby mitigating its effect. If, for instance, I doubt another's word, people who know the speaker can vouch for him or her, thereby reducing my doubt to a manageable and therefore, acceptable level. Unfortunately, others are less apt to be able to eliminate doubt about our own misgivings and our understanding of ourselves.

Just because others are "less apt" to be of use does not mean that they can't be helpful resources. Because doubt involves some kind of decision, its resolution, decision-making, rests within the individual. This is often a forgotten fact. Not to decide is, after all, a decision to procrastinate the making of another decision. This is where doubt is helpful. There are times when a decision ought not to be made, when there are reasonable, acceptable, and important reasons to not proceed upon a certain course of action. In fact, one might be well-advised to not make a decision when there is doubt. Doubt is often a warning sign, if not to refrain from acting, then to at least delay action until the doubt is resolved, which in many cases, means that it is significantly reduced, rather than totally eliminated.

The point here is to recognize the presence of doubt, to accept that one is indeed deciding not to act because of it, and then to begin a process that increases the level of certainty about the person, action, or relationship so that one feels safe in proceeding. As long as doubt is strong enough to overpower our feelings of safety, it needs to be given credence.

The challenge here is to be able to articulate what one doubts, to make those doubts specific so that they may be specifically addressed. Like fear, the expression of doubt, either by writing about it in a journal or by voicing it to a friend, counselor, or mentor can be the first step in reducing its power. Here is where we must recognize our own part in the doubt. To remain doubtful without taking steps to reduce it is, in fact, to decide to stay in doubt. It is your life and you are free to do as you wish, but you will live with the outcome of that decision. It is important to avoid thinking of oneself as a victim. We do this when we project that the cause of our doubt lies with someone else. It is our responsibility to ascertain the truth, to eliminate our doubt by research. Not to do so indicates that we are choosing to remain doubtful and are refusing to make responsible, that is well-informed, decisions.

Most doubts, happily, can be overcome simply by referring to others who have more experience, either by reading pertinent literature or by consulting trustworthy players. Many doubts, too, are based on erroneous expectations and the simple act of clarifying expectations will lessen the doubt. Many slave-applicants, for instance, doubt that they will be able to do a certain activity. Let me use fisting as an example. Slave-applicant, Tom, wants to serve a master, but refuses to do so because he doubts that he could ever be fisted. He may, in fact, fear such an action and therefore doubts that he can do it. In reality, his prospective master may have no desire whatsoever to fist his slave. In this case, the master-to-be's assurance will go a long way to alleviate the slave-to-be's doubt, since fisting, in this scenario, is not a consideration, even if the slave's doubt is.

Because so many of our ideas about M/s relationships are based on fiction, it is natural to construct expectations and scenarios that are highly doubtful. Nonetheless, we believe these inaccuracies and allow them to foster fear of the future and doubt about our own adequacy in the situation. The facts, and only the facts, will clear this up for us, allowing us to proceed on the path which will bring our fantasies to fruition. Use reality, not fantasy, to resolve your doubts and you will find yourself living the kind of life you seek.

Having gotten thus far, you can decide on some course of action.

Small steps will reduce the risks as well. You don't have to go whole hog in this process. Use easy actions, ones that demand little expense or exposure to test the waters. No one says you can't try it as an experiment, the results of which will help give you more information and hence dispel more fear and doubt. There are, of course, psychological tools that will help you overcome fear. Counseling, meditation, and relaxation are among them. These are acceptable courses of action, as are attending seminars, consulting experts, and reading books.

Eventually, you will have to act, even if your action is mostly inaction. It's your life and your choice. I would only caution that if you keep on doing what you've always done, you'll keep on getting what you've always gotten. Creating your M/s relationship is going to take work; so, you might as well start now, lest the price of this book be spent for naught.

There is the possibility of a wonderful world awaiting you as master or as slave. Mutual empowerment is the real goal here, not defeat of one or the other. Leather is meant to be a win-win situation. As for Charles, next time — and I hope there'll be a next time — I'll have those cards ready. More than that, I'll make sure that I express my thanks and my affection before I fall asleep. After all, I want to succeed as much as the next guy.

The 24/7 Dilemma

During one of the four workshops I once gave in St. Louis (those folks know how to get a lot of work out of their presenters), a woman, who is also slave to her husband, asked how one remains submissive all the time. The question really boils down to: "How do we live 24/7 in a real world?" That is one that we all face. There's usually no problem with being kinky in the bedroom with the door closed, but how do you stay in that state at work, in front of your children or parents, or when the vanilla world is watching you?

Similarly, how do we transit from one mode to the other without "coming down?" How do we incorporate our kinkiness into our lives so that we can be ourselves without becoming outcast?

Some might answer the question with bold statements about "coming out," becoming public. Radical and iconoclastic, they would say damn what other people think. Easy words, to be sure, but they don't reflect the consequences that flaunting and rebelling will incur.

Certainly, some of us can be, and are, very public about how we live. I'm out to my parents and my children. Though I don't go into specifics unless directly asked, my colleagues at work know what I write and some of them have some vague ideas about my sex life. My closest colleagues in the teachers' union know about my relationships and my books. A few have actually asked to read them.

I'm a loud mouth extrovert who wears his heart on his sleeve. I can't keep a secret about myself very well, though I am good at keeping others' confidential information. I've prospered by being out, but in all truth, I have, at times, paid the price of living parts of my private life in public. To wit, my parents have never, and won't, visit my home since my Dad is afraid of what he will see. Likewise, I am sure I have been passed over when it comes to getting a new job and some men have avoided dating me because I'm "Jack Rinella."

Nevertheless, there are ways to stay kinky with discretion. After all, I don't flaunt my sexuality and sadomasochism in my computer classes. Strangers would never suspect what I write or how Patrick and I play. In public, my slave and I look like any other two men. At the Masonic Lodge, where I am a member, I participate in the same way as the others and there are few, very few, references to my writing, my public speaking, and my sex life.

My daughters know that Patrick is my slave, but they have never seen him naked, kiss my feet, or bound and flogged. They don't have to. Though my daughter (an adult in her own right) reads my columns she doesn't usually comment on them. All of that, I think, is fine. There is a time and a place for everything. Discretion is as necessary as public display, privacy as important as publicity.

How, then, shall we live 24/7? How is a mother a slave to her husband in front of her children? How is a person Dominant in front of his or her right-wing boss? How can we be kinky when being kinky means ostracism, persecution, or consequences we can't afford to endure? The answer is certainly individualized. There are no simple solutions, no one size fits all. There are, though, principles that can guide us. First and foremost, we must be ready to accept the consequences of our actions. Like it or not, there will be consequences and they should be weighed carefully before we act. Sometimes, they must be suffered, as that is the right thing to do.

Often, though, they may be easily avoided with silence, with euphemisms, or with discretion — which my handy dictionary defines as: "the quality of being discreet; circumspection; Freedom to act or judge on one's own." If that definition leaves something to desire, we only need to see what the word discreet means: "Having or showing a judicious reserve in one's speech or behavior; prudent," which is: "wise in handling practical matters; exercising good judgment or common sense."

Note that all of these definitions refer to outward actions. The trick, therefore, is to stay in the headspace, while we appear to be physically in another space. We look like businessmen, sales clerks, teachers, mothers, or sons to our eighty year-old parents, while we know that we are kinky sadists or groveling subs.

The mother, who has trouble being mother and slave in front of her daughters, can own her slavery as wife and mother, remembering that being a good mother means being a good slave to her husband. Mothering, or any other activity for that matter, becomes a manifestation of submission when we remember that we are doing it because we have chosen to do it and why we have made that choice. Once again, I might remind her that submissive doesn't necessarily mean passive.

Most of us, hell all of us, have to live in a real world. Though I have no statistics, I am certain that the vast majority of kinky folks are kinky in scenes, not every minute of the day, every day of the week. Patrick eats at the table with me, not from a dish on the floor. When I sleep, I dominate no one, and quite frankly, I don't want to be waken to be asked if my sub can take a piss.

Part of this discussion revolves around the idea of real. The scenes we enjoy are real and so are the chores, the careers, and the mundane day to day lives that allow us the moments we call scenes. Stop living the mundane and you will soon have no resources to enjoy the scenes.

The answer, then, is to see the connectedness in all we do: that job, family, sleep, and the rest, empower us to be kinky. Cease living a real life and you will soon cease living a kinky one, too. The answer is in the way we perceive what we do. As the dictionary says, a person has the "Freedom to act or judge on one's own." If that freedom means we are submissive, we can know we are submissive, and in fact be so, without others knowing to whom, or even that, we are being so.

The slave-mother can appear to be in control because she is controlling in obedience to her master-husband. The dominant can do as his boss asks because he has chosen to work for the boss. In both cases, what is constant is that one acts as one chooses, even if the logic of the choices is not readily apparent to those who see the actions.

So, Patrick calls me "Sir," and those in the know think that he's a good slave. Those not so informed think he just does it because he's a polite Southern gentleman, that the Sir he calls me is the same as the Sir he calls my father. It's not, of course, but my dad doesn't need to know.

Everyday Living[†]

A reader named Bob once wrote me a letter asking: "Could you write about a typical evening with Patrick from the time you get home from work? Maybe it would give me — and others — some new ideas.

[†] Let me caution you that this section illustrates life in my home. Your life in your home may well be very different.

I need to do something to spice up my activity with my slave. Evenings are becoming too predictable."

Long-term relationships run the risk of becoming stagnant. Avoiding such a trap, if that's what you think it is, takes communication with your partner. There is no secret formula to keeping the fires hot, except that you have to remember to keep stoking them. So, what is my usual life like? I'm afraid that it's pretty predictable, though that is not a complaint. We are who we are and most often, just do what we usually do. Here's the blow by blow, so speak.

I usually wake up first. Patrick is sleeping on the futon next to my bed. He prefers that and has never wanted to sleep with me. If I am horny (four out of seven mornings a week), I'll reach my foot from under the covers, jostling him until he wakes. Then, I throw back the covers, spread my legs and tell him to suck. That is followed by his making me coffee.

Twice a week, I have to leave early to teach. Patrick doesn't start work until 10 AM; so, he can get a later start. On other days, as a self-employed writer, I am home most of the day, except when I have to go for errands, like going to the bank or visiting the library. In any case, I am most often home in the mid-afternoon. My day is filled with thinking, writing, answering e-mail, researching, resting, errands and lots of chores that consume one's time, like balancing checkbooks and paying bills. I am the financial one in the house.

Come five or so, I begin to relax, usually with a vodka on the rocks, with hand-stuffed (by Patrick) anchovy olives. Sometimes I wait for Patrick to come home to make it for me. At other times, I do it myself. If the supply of olives is low, I leave the bottle out so he can stuff me a few. It's a job he doesn't like.

By 6:30 PM or so, Patrick is home and begins cooking dinner. I often sit in the kitchen and we talk as he does it. Upon arriving home, Patrick kneels on the floor, kisses each foot or shoe and recites, "Sir, please train me to please you, Sir," or whatever his mantra is at the time. I answer, "I'll try." He then goes and strips, as that is his uniform. He often wears socks to keep his feet warm. If the house is cold, he may ask (or just presume) to keep his clothes on. Who wants a cold slave?

The two of us have dinner together at the dining room table, like any household anywhere, except for the nudity and the chain collar. Of course, it is also noticeable that I don't lift a finger for anything except to feed myself. From that, you can correctly surmise that Patrick does all the meal planning, shopping, cooking, and cleaning. So, yes, I just sit on the couch, and watch him work and serve. He is my slave, after all. On the other hand, he takes pride in his service. Patrick is especially proud of his cooking and loves to do it. Happily, he is good at it, very good.

By now, it's 8:30 PM, or so, and I'm ready for bed; so, I go off into the bedroom, where Patrick has already turned down the covers, lowered the lights, and, if it's cool, turned on the electric heater. I often turn on a video and watch it half-heartedly, while waiting for him to join me.

When the kitchen is clean, or sooner (if I yell for him), he comes in. He kneels on the side of the bed and awaits my orders. Often, we will begin just by talking, sometimes we cuddle, or I'll just tell him to suck my dick. Some nights, I play with a trick or an applicant instead of him; when visitors leave, I often then call for him.

Though Patrick doesn't like the idea that I watch the clock, a usual night of sex takes anywhere from 20 to 90 minutes. One night, it might be fucking, another bondage, another clothespins or mummification, another a lot of ass-play or slapping or cock and ball torture. I am very eclectic in my tastes, and obviously have attention deficit disorder, as I don't do any one thing for very long. I think Patrick thinks it's more like musical sex chairs than romance.

Needless to say, the bedroom is supplied with a few toys. A greater assortment is in the dungeon in the basement, which I use two or three nights a week. My favorites include butt plugs (especially the inflatable kind), clothespins, ace bandages, candles for atmosphere and dripping (but not often, as it's too messy), lots of rope and I mean lots. I have a rim seat that gets used more often than not (for finishing me off, so to speak). If I'm going to get more rambunctious, I'll go downstairs since there are a great number of hooks for bondage, a sling, and most of my whips and crops. What more could a master want?**

Finally, I shoot my load and lay still. When I eventually move, Patrick covers my cum and my cock with a towel then covers me with the sheet and blanket and I'm gone for a while into dreamland. He will then go do whatever he wants. It's not unusual for me to sleep for an hour or so, then yell for him to come back into the bedroom for round two. At other times, I've been known to sleep for several hours and then wake him up in the middle of the night.

Herein, then, are some of the clues to keeping the fires burning well. We communicate a great deal with one another to find out what we want and need and to make sure we're both getting it. Secondly, I am eclectic; so, we do and try a lot of different things, not every night, but often enough. Visiting events and the vendors that attend them offer new ideas and new toys. Thirdly, the bedroom is well-stocked for play, though in past years, we've actually started in the living room, in front of the fireplace (when we had one), fairly often.

** The answer, of course, is additional slaves.

174

In any case, you don't find much boredom in the Rinella household. What else do you want to know?

Rituals

One of the more noticeable characteristics of the master/ slave relationship is that it is often marked by formal, ritualistic, and/or signifying actions and tokens, such as a collar, or the fact that the slave stands with hands behind his or her back, behind and to one side of the master. As in practically everything else, you're not going to find any "standard" ritual for expressing the M/s relationship among its practitioners.

What you will find is that most masters prescribe certain actions as the way their slave will acknowledge their slavery. Masters, too, have usual ways of expressing their mastery. One of the popular ways that each demonstrate their respective mastery and slavery is through protocols, which I have already discussed, and through rituals.

In this case, a ritual is best described as: "a detailed method or procedure faithfully or regularly followed." In our subculture, some of which we call protocol is, in fact, ritual. Other practices may be best called manners.

One of the times where rituals are most often seen, though they may not always be seen in public, is when the slave greets the master. Commonly known as "presenting," it usually takes the form of kneeling when the slave enters the master's presence after an absence or when the master returns after a period of time and enters the slave's presence. Some masters train their slaves to do more than kneel and await an order to rise.

My slave, Patrick, for instance, kneels, kisses each of my feet, recites a short phrase (which we call a mantra), and remains bowed before me until I bid him rise. Over time, the specific phrase has changed. Initially, it was something like "I am here to serve you, Sir." Later I changed it to, "Please train me to please you, Sir," and as of the writing of this book it is "I am your fuck bitch, Sir."

Our sex life contains a few rituals as well, such that, for instance, when I stretch out my hand and snap my finger, Patrick knows that this is a sign for him to put his testicles in the palm of my hand. Rituals may also be developed to begin a scene, at the start of a meal, or upon rising in the morning. In master/slave relationships with more of a spiritual bend, there may be rituals concerning prayer, as well.

Dress and Markings

Masters often take pleasure not only in a slave's actions, but in their appearance, as well. Therefore, one will find that each master has a given preference for the slave to wear a collar, to be tattooed, branded, or scarred in a certain way, or to wear a distinctive garb or hairstyle. And, yes, these preferences vary greatly — as if I had to write that line one more time!

It is interesting to note that the slave collar is rather ubiquitous in our subculture and that the greater number of collars are rather discreet. Some, in fact, easily pass as nothing more than a piece of fancy jewelry. Patrick wears a light, stainless steel chain purchased from a nautical supply company. It fits loosely around his neck and is fastened with a small brass lock, the key to which I keep. Honestly, though, the lock has been on for so long that the key probably no longer works and, indeed, I would be hard-pressed to find it quickly. In any case, it doesn't set off metal detectors at airports, causes no skin irritation, and in an emergency, could be easily removed with a pair of pliers. Another master has his slaves wear distinctive uniform-like shirts; some masters enjoy having their slaves wear silks and laces to make them look like Arabian slaves; others require their male slaves to keep their heads or bodies shaven.

Although wearing a collar generally signifies that the wearer is under another's control, the sad fact is that they are too often worn as a fashion statement. I write this only as a warning so you'll know not to make any assumptions about the person wearing a collar, and to suggest that even though you consider yourself slave material, you not put a collar on yourself. It's always safer to ask the wearer what the collar means, rather than to come to an erroneous conclusion.

In my personal practice, there are three kinds of collars. In the first case, I use a collar, usually a leather one that's simply buckled on, as part of a scene. It defines, for the time, the kind of relationship that I and my temporary partner will have for the duration of our play. When we decide to enter into more serious training, I'll offer the applicant a training collar for a specific length of time — a weekend, week, or month. In this case and the next, I use the light stainless steel collar mentioned above.

Lastly, of course, is the full slave collar like the one that Patrick wears. Many masters, it should be noted, adhere to a similar usage. Additionally, you will find a wide range of "dress up" collars made of leather, silver, and chain mail.

As a personal note, I would like to remind all my readers that collars are usually the property of the dominant and ought to be returned when the relationship is terminated. If it's not obvious, I write this paragraph as a man who has lost way too many collars.

Permanent body modifications ought to be done only after the relationship has withstood the test of time. I had a professional piercer put a guiche[††] into Patrick after we were together for some three years. In 2004, after we had been together more than eight years, I had a tattoo placed on his right ass cheek. It is a circle about two inches in diameter with the word "slave" boldly place in the center. Inside the circumference are the words, in a smaller size, "Property of Jack Rinella."

Most masters agree that those seeking slavery ought not to mark themselves in anticipation of slavery, but rather that they should present themselves to their master as a rather "clean slate," so that the master will have the pleasure of marking them as he or she sees fit.[‡‡] On the other hand, if you already have tats, rings, or some other body modification, I certainly wouldn't worry about it.

The Mutual Need for Expression

What the preceding section illustrates is that we all have a desire, perhaps even a need, to find ways to express that which is within. Let me remind you that the first and foremost characteristic of the slave, meaning he or she who demonstrates servitude through actions, is that he or she has the right attitude. Let me restate it in bold letters: **Having the right attitude is what's most important.**

There is something intrinsic to human nature that we want to express to the world that which we feel and think. Hence we find ways to do so.

Unfortunately, the master/slave relationship isn't exactly acceptable in modern society. We all know that to broadcast our rather unique and certainly, alternative lifestyle, in a willy-nilly fashion, will only cause grief. In this instance, "Discretion is the better part of valor." Therefore, there are pubic, private, and familial expressions that we use to express our relationship, and they vary with the amount of privacy, understanding, and acceptance available to us.

Considering Reality —
Family, Friends, and Employer

In an ideal world, there would be no secrets and no need for privacy. Tolerance and acceptance would be universal. Fear and reprisal would be nonexistent. As you may have noticed, we live on a planet in a universe where not all is friendly, helpful, or virtuous. That certainly explains the need for discretion.

One might wish that we could all be ourselves in every place and

†† A small surgical steel ring in his skin between his scrotum and his anus.

‡‡ The master's ability to mark may be limited by what's been negotiated.

every time, but such is not the case. Therefore rules and expectations need to be adjusted accordingly. Simply put, the best guideline is to use one's common sense and if you don't have common sense, then ask a few respected members of your kinky community what they would do.

Another valuable guideline is to "KISS," that is "keep it simple, stupid." Complexity is generally unnecessary and simplicity certainly has its advantages. Remembering that such is the case will make your life and that of your master or slave much easier and happier.

Domestic Violence

I've changed his name to Andy in order to protect him. Protecting one another is an important part of being in the BDSM community. In fact, being active in a real time and place BDSM community is itself a form of protection. It's for that reason that I always suggest that anyone searching to be part of an SM relationship, first be part of one of the many kinky communities you'll find across our country.

We are, of course, not a single community, so much as a community of communities that shares our love and practice of kink — even though our kinks vary as widely as our expressions of gender, sexuality, and organization. Some of us are liberals, some conservative; some religious, some not; many are heterosexual, some gay, and most (whether they practice it or not) are bisexual. Nevertheless, most of us share a belief that what it is that we do needs to be (in some fashion) safe, sane, and consensual. I trust my Risk Aware Consensual Kink (RACK) friends will understand that I am not discounting their alternative expression of the fact that we do our best to avoid both injury and non-consensual play.

The telling line in Andy's e-mail is this: "Jack, I can't see that BDSM is anything more than systematized, glorified child abuse in a different form." Having given emphasis to his most important statement, let's look at the heart of his communication to me:

> I do know that I was an incest victim and it is the poor self-image, expectation of abuse, and generally victimized (plus craving more, because that's the dirty little secret of incest — the sub always likes it) mindset that later led me to try and become slave.
>
> I did okay at being a slave, Jack, except I kept expecting the top to behave according to some kind of moral principles and none of the three men did so. In fact, that is exactly in keeping with the parental-abuser mode, since there isn't a parent in the world who does abuse his or her children and then thinks of ways to do it morally.
>
> Jack, I can't see that BDSM is anything more than systematized, glorified child abuse in a different form. Got any answers for

me?[§§]

Now I am certainly not one to avoid giving an answer. It should be obvious that I have an opinion on most everything. On the other hand I am not competent to advise Andy how to solve his problem. I am not a therapist and have no intention of becoming one. I already have a Masters degree and don't want to spend another three years and more than $10,000 to get one.

Whether we consider the problem of child abuse or domestic violence, we need to note the differences between those two evils and BDSM. For a proper delineation of those differences, I refer you to:

http://www.nlaidvproject.us

— a website of the National Leather Association's Domestic Violence Project.

Domestic violence (DV) is not an easy topic to discuss, in so far as it can bring up a lot of complicated emotions in all of us: pain, shame, betrayal, guilt, or fear. But we need to understand and recognize the signs of abuse, the cycle of abuse (build-up, confrontation, and honeymoon), and know what resources are available to us. Anyone can be subject to abuse: a person's size, gender, or specific sex role (e.g. top/bottom, butch/femme), is irrelevant. Domestic Violence is a pattern of intentional intimidation for the purpose of dominating, coercing, or isolating another without his/her consent. Abuse tends to be cyclical in nature and escalates over time.

Notice, then, some of the distinguishing marks of DV. It is non-consensual and cyclical. Occurrences of DV are followed by remorse, fear, shame, and a complete lack of the pleasure, comfort, and satisfaction that a healthy SM scene demonstrates. The abuser doesn't negotiate, he or she intimidates.

What then, can I tell Andy? First off, I would talk about his self-image and the fact that healthy BDSM and healthy tops and bottoms (including healthy masters and slaves) recognize that we all have an obligation to support each other in developing and maintaining a healthy self-image. It is as simple as that. We need to actively give positive reinforcement to one another, the kind that encourages all players to realize their high self-worth, no matter what their sexual preferences, proclivities, and fetishes.

Next, I would remind Andy that his self-image is exactly that: HIS self-image. If his motivation in being involved in a master/slave relationship is, in fact, based on a poor self-image, then he needs to know that that kind of relationship is not for him. BDSM is neither therapy nor escape nor abuse. As you will read in chapter nine, slaves

§§ Unpublished email received on December 4, 2004.

in successful relationships are in fact, confident, strong, and self-assured.

There certainly are survivors of child abuse and domestic violence in our midst, but the ones I've met are people who have come to healthy terms with their past and understand the difference between abuse and pleasurable, consensual SM.

Though some subs may think they like abuse, I am not sure I can agree with the assessment that they all share that "dirty little secret." If one does feel that way, that is definitely a good reason to seek competent counseling, as well as to exit (or don't enter) the DV relationship. Unfortunately, no one can pull anyone out of a relationship that he doesn't want to end. After all, "poor self-image, expectation of abuse, and a generally victimized "mindset" are never, either singly or jointly, valid reasons to seek slavery. There are, of course, good reasons to submit to another, but they relate to personal empowerment, pleasure, and the desire to serve. Look at the real slaves in our midst and you will find healthy, happy, self-confident, and strong individuals committed to their masters in a healthy, happy, and positive relationship.

Andy, I am sorry that your expectations were never met by the masters who you encountered. I can't say why that is the case, as I neither know your expectations nor theirs, or both sides of the story. I can say, though, that quite possibly you didn't enter into the relationship with full disclosure on both sides, frankly stating your expectations, revealing your past, and acknowledging your need for release from the victimization and abuse of your childhood.

To be honest, I encounter men and women who seek slavery for what appears to be the wrong reasons all the time. Like other healthy masters, I am rather quick to debunk their myths about what I can and can't do and what I will and won't do. Frankly, I will correct every negative statement uttered by a submissive. I will remind submissives that they are good people, beautiful and capable. I will do my best to back my words with actions that support, encourage, and affirm their very high worth as humans. I ask you not to judge all of us by the examples of those who are not what we aspire to be.

For those searching for a master, I would add that they ought to be sure the man or woman they seek is safe, sane, and believe that the M/s relationship was meant to empower and encourage — never meant to demean or belittle.

This e-mail and these words bring to mind exactly why our individual communities are so very important. It is invariably the "lone ranger" who is the abuser and the victimizer. Our communities do not and will not condone abuse and violence, and we are generally quick to aid those caught in its ugly cycles.

Once again, we are not the experts. If abuse and domestic violence plague your life, or if they ever did, I urge you to find a competent counselor and to learn how high a value you really have. Good luck. Feel free to contact me (and not just Andy, but anyone) if I can be of help.

I would also refer you to: The National Domestic Violence Hotline at 1-800-799-SAFE (7233) or 1-800-787-3224 (TTY). Their address is PO Box 161810, Austin, Texas 78716 and their website is at http://www.ndvh.org.

Financial Considerations

When they say, "It's not the money. It's the principle of the thing," you can be sure that it's the money. At least, that's what my mother taught me. Everyone has some issue to deal with, usually centered around health, finances, or relationships.

Over the years, fiction has fed my imagination. Time and time again, stories about "The Network," slavery rings, or mountain men selling their sons to cowboys have fueled my mind with fantasies that made me stiff. In his series of books on the Network, John Preston laid out an elaborate, hidden culture of wealth and sex, where men and women (always the best looking and well educated types) sold themselves into servitude for large, but never disclosed, amounts of money, systematically deposited in secret, numbered bank accounts in banks on some unnamed Caribbean Island.

Nice work if you can get it.

I've never found a shred of evidence that just such a system exists. To the contrary, I've found that the vast numbers of Leather players are no different from the rest of the world when it comes to cash on hand. As I scan the Leather landscape, most slave-applicants are broke, most masters far from able to support their imaginations with adequate funding. That appraisal was seconded by Master Panman. When I talked with him about "brokering," he quickly pointed out that no one was going to pay the thousands of dollars such an arrangement would cost.

I once negotiated with a man in Los Angeles, who couldn't find a master in that wide open town. He was in debt to the syndicate, also know as the Mafia. His, apparently, real desire to serve was completely stymied by a "bill collector" who regularly met him in the parking lot of the factory where he worked for minimum wages. By the time the collector "cashed" his check, there was nothing left past mere living expenses.

Not every form of slavery is sexual, consensual, or enjoyable. I figured that for between 4,000 and 5,000 dollars, I could have bought the debt and owned the boy. Most writers, myself included, don't have that kind of money to throw around. So ended the negotiations. As you can see, slave searching quickly enters into stark realism when the discussion turns to money.

Let me continue the discussion with an excerpt from my "Expectations and Regulations concerning Voluntary Servitude:"

> Finances. Upon entry into servitude, the slave will turn practical and actual (but not legal) control of his personal resources over to the Master for administration.
>
> Assets will remain the property of the slave. Nothing in this section is meant to infer that the Master is using the relationship for his own aggrandizement. Similarly this is not a 'free ride' for the slave. The Master will administer the slave's finances in such a way as to increase their value and provide for the slave's present and future needs.
>
> The slave will support himself and provide for the Master's pleasure and prosperity. The Master will not accept the role of providing for the slave — as that would in fact make him the slave's slave, a role the Master is not willing to accept. As the Master's property the slave will not be allowed to become a drain on the Master's finances, but rather an asset to them.¶¶

For starters, there is the underlying premise that relationships ought to be entered into slowly. The so-called master who requires immediate full financial disclosure and the slave-wannabe, who expects a sugar daddy, are both dreaming. Likewise, powers of attorney are not instruments of domination and submission, especially when you've never met the person who asks for it. Financial entanglements ought to be made with extreme caution and only after any relationship has begun to pass the test of time. As I made clear earlier, professional advice from a lawyer or accountant is not uncalled for. As easily as Patrick has fit into my household, there have been difficulties with finances.

Patrick came to me shortly after leaving another master, one who had taken advantage of his trust. In the end, Patrick lost several thousand dollars. The loss may have been larger if Patrick hadn't sensed some chicanery underfoot and called a halt to the process. Accordingly, Patrick felt it necessary when he moved in to set aside a store of cash for himself, of which I had no knowledge. It was "insurance" against the possibility that I would leave him high, dry, and broke. I strongly advise those considering master/slave relationships to consider alternatives and to test their commitments before tying the financial knot. Divorce courts are ample testimony to the problems of disassembling households,

¶¶ See Appendix C.

but they won't consider any relationship, except that of heterosexual marriage. It's not that the master and slave don't need to come to an understanding about money. Rather, they need to come up with a realistic one.

Slaves can't function without bus fare, parking fees, and lunch money. Monthly expenses for food, housing, medical care, transportation, clothing, and entertainment aren't slight. The slave who expects his master or mistress to care for him or her is delusional. The master who thinks that owning a slave is without cost is living with his head in very strange clouds.

What kind of guidelines might we expect to use? How about: "Take it slowly, one day at a time?" Over the course of months, whatever changes and commingling of funds is necessary will become evident. In addition to a reasonable pace, honesty needs to be maintained. Understand how much things really cost, know who is actually responsible, and plan accordingly.

It's nice to think that Patrick slavishly bestows his paycheck on me. The implications for that, though, are that I'm stuck with his bills too. If I lay claim to his money, he can lay claim to my being responsible. If he lives under my roof, he becomes obligated to help pay for that roof.

There are ways to cope with questions of finance. What it takes to arrive at financial answers is honest and realistic planning. Discuss the implications of commitment. How does it affect debt, savings, and day to day living? No master can be there with an open wallet every minute of the day. No slave can expect that his or her master will bail her out every time a bill comes due.

If you're negotiating, ask about budgeting, saving for the future, and eliminating debt. If the slave won't be working outside the home, how will he or she be supported? Know what contingencies there are for emergencies, for comfort, and for the future.

I know a man, now very successful and very independent, who, as a young adult, was kept caged and naked in his master's apartment. That arrangement fell apart when the master suddenly died and the slave was cast out by the estate. Penniless, uneducated, without any work history, it was only when a few friends of the late master came to the slave's financial aid that a totally impossible situation was resolved.

The End

Even the healthiest and happiest relationships will end. Both masters and slaves have been left bereft of their partner through death, career changes, change of heart, and a myriad of reasons that bring about a breakup. I am reminded of, for instance, a loving master/slave couple that was devastated by the slave's unexpected infection with pneumonia.

The master had suggested on many occasions that the slave be tested for HIV and the slave consistently refused. By the time the pneumonia was diagnosed (as was AIDS), it was too late. Within the month, the slave was dead, leaving a grieving master, who had to cope with the slave's unsympathetic family. Since there was no will, the master now had legal and financial trauma while he additionally had to deal with his own recently diagnosed infection.

Since this is a book about becoming a slave, you're probably not interested in reading about ending the master/slave relationship. Yet end it will.

Statistics, quite frankly, show that most master/slave relationships don't last more than three or four months, though there certainly are many that have survived as long, and longer, than ours. This is not to cast aspersion on the nature of D/s relationships, as in all probability, many other very vanilla relationships have the same measly track record. Once again, our relationships are human relationships, and as such, are simply mortal. In the joy of meeting and the excitement of building the M/s relationship, it is very easy to ignore the long-term future, since procrastination is a very easy practice.

Like beginnings, ends should be undertaken slowly, with counseling, planning, and mutual consideration of what is fair and just. Unfortunately, newly coupled dominants and submissives probably don't want to consider the end of their relationship and those who are contemplating just such a move, are most often either too distraught or too angry to be "fair and just." My advice is to seek guidance about separating — long before you need it — and to plan accordingly.

Dreams of servitude might get you off, but the piper must be paid. Plan now to have the wherewithal necessary.

Patrick Relfects: Stuff, Tips and Tricks for Success
Fear

Fear comes in many forms and touches many aspects of our lives. After I discovered erotic dominance and submission, the power of D/s frightened me, not the control, but the intensity and rightness of it. It took ten years, with a little dabbling here and there, before I could begin to take my first active steps to explore what it really had to offer me.

One form of fear, as Sir mentioned, is of failure. For me it manifested itself as a fear of being laughed at, that I was foolish enough to take fiction seriously, to learn that something I'd invested ten years dreaming about was fiction, a prop for getting laid. I was afraid of being ridiculed.

There is the fear of giving up independence for control, of being taken further than we are ready for, of not finding fulfillment, of being "found out" by family and friends and employers, and of being different than what is perceived as "normal" by society. It takes many forms, and it stifles us, and keeps us afraid to grow.

Safer Sex

It amazes me that there is so much resistance, especially among Gay men, of practicing safer sex. We invest so much energy in image, in protecting our investments, in securing our property, in enhancing our careers and professions, yet so often people are willing to put the benefactor of that energy, their bodies, at risk.

The other amazement I have is how much fear there is, again more prevalent among Gay men, of involving yourself with someone who is HIV positive. Instead they limit themselves to those who say they are negative with the misguided notion that they are safer playing with and having sex with them. The reality is that people often assume they are negative because they are afraid to find out their status, don't want to effectively educate themselves in order to stay that way, and assume that someone infected with the virus is reckless and unsafe and a risk.

There is no better way to contract sexually transmitted diseases than through denial. As someone who is negative but well-informed and who is not the least bit afraid to play with someone who is positive, I can say that no one is going to be more conscious of not infecting someone then someone who intimately understands the ramifications of doing so. All you do by practicing this prejudice is lessen your chances of finding your own happiness.

The 24/7 dilemma

Sir's description of our typical daily routine will come across a bit mundane, even if we weren't master and slave. Neither of us enjoys going out a great deal and we aren't watchers of television. He goes to bed earlier but tends to get up earlier as well. Sex and play probably happens more than is typical, (Hey, not going out or watching television allows a lot more time for this), but the fact is that much of our time together is routine.

Those who've not been in a 24/7 relationship usually focus their thinking on the sex and the bondage but in longer-term relationships the reality is that those are only minor portions of a typical day.

For a planned weekend when you are first meeting, the master or mistress will generally put aside everything they can and focus his or her time and energy on exploring who you are and what you can do together. There's a raised level of energy and excitement over the prospect of having you there. There is the expectation of hot sex and a good time. Playtime will be better planned, more frequent, and more intense.

A special intensity surrounds a short term M/s experience. Time takes over the scene and encourages eroticism. The excitement and pleasure that both the dominant and submissive take away from a successful short encounter can be very powerful. The limited time enhances everything that happens and a submissive can let him or herself go whole-heartedly into the experience and take it as far as they can because of the knowledge that there is a definite end time. The dominant often tries to cram more variety into the experience and play with wild abandon (to the extent of the negotiated limits), especially if there is a definite chemistry between them, and this adds to the energy and endorphins. Short encounters tend to be a cornucopia of pleasure for both players, whether it is an evening, a weekend, or a week. And then it ends, and they take away from it feelings that tend to be magnified when they think back on them, and it drives their fantasy life.

If the relationship evolves into a longer-term relationship that same kind of intensity is there in the beginning. Much like young love there is freshness, passion, and a general dreaminess about it. Little by little, though, things begin to occupy your master's time and energy once you are there for an extended period of time. Everyday life pokes its ugly head into the relationship and demands to be handled. Bills have to be paid, grocery shopping needs to be done, the house need to be cleaned, and laundry needs doing; careers or jobs take up significant amounts of time and deplete available energy. The focus is less on passion and more on maintenance, and this is necessary, though not always understood.

Just as man cannot live on bread alone we can't survive only on passion. The energy expended needs to be replenished, and replenishing it can be a bit mundane. Life is different with an on-going relationship and those who don't understand this will find themselves wondering what has happened to their fantasy.

That's the 24/7 dilemma and understanding it allows you to understand what is happening as it happens, and to plan how to successfully wade through that phase of the relationship. It's also important to understand that masters, for all they know, don't necessarily understand this dynamic either. It doesn't come with the territory.

Public Exposure

Just prior to becoming Sir's slave I was in a brief, four-month relationship. The relationship ended for a variety of reasons and one of the minor ones was that during that time my master was obsessed with attracting attention. He tried to make every part of our lifestyle in the small Texas panhandle city where we lived something to be stared at and talked about. He had me keep my head shaved except for a small lock of hair on the back of my head that he wanted me to grow into a ponytail. He pierced my right ear and had me wear a large ring with a hanging ball in it. Clothes were generally well-worn and ragged and he insisted that I wear a wide, thick, black leather collar in public that had multiple rings on it, usually with a leash hanging from it. He would take it off around the house but we never went anywhere without my wearing it. He looked like a worn out, poverty-stricken Willie Nelson, with hair at least as long, and he never had me park anywhere close to where we were going in order to attract as much attention as possible. If I had been a teenager it might have been different, but at age 39 I was really a spectacle.

I endured it like a good slave but it made for some uncomfortable situations. To make matters worse, when he was with me, if anyone gave me more than a passing glance he would make a further spectacle by being loud and badgering towards them.

I've found that in general most people adopt an attitude of live and let live that allows for a lot of diversity, even in a small town, but when it becomes an "In your face" kind of thing I think it's out of place and doesn't help the relationship or the community as a whole.

For instance, I wear a chain collar with a small brass lock. In general the lock hangs just below my collar line, not because I'm trying to hide it, but because that's where it ends up after I put on my shirt. Sir doesn't require that it be visible but at times it flops out and I don't think twice about it. When that happens and people notice it I do get some odds looks and occasionally a comment but nothing really out of place or offensive. Sometimes people ask about it and my reply is "Someone very special gave it to me." The response from people has never been negative and is generally along the lines of "That's nice", or "That person must be very special", or "It must be nice to have someone caring about you". I've never been given a hard time about it. This "don't scare the natives" behavior should work well for most anyone most anywhere.

At events where our community comes together one can be more public and at ease about showing that you are master and slave couple and I heartily recommend that you take time to be so. If you are not in a full-time relationship yet, attending an event will give you opportunity to experience how others live their lifestyle as well as perhaps aid in finding your future master. If you are in a relationship you and your master will find acceptance, support and camaraderie, a secure environment where you can relax and enjoy who you are and even learn a thing or two. Appendix E lists some events and resources beneficial to those interested in D/s relationships and I encourage you to check them out.

Keep in mind, though, that it can be just as bad to be overly concerned about what people will think or find out. The fear and stress generated by being overly paranoid about being found out is just as unhealthy, both health-wise and for the relationship. Most often people don't give things a second thought so your obsessing over it is unnecessary. You and your master will adopt a lifestyle that fits you and the community in which you live and you shouldn't have to keep looking over your shoulder to ensure that you aren't revealing too much.

Friends, Family, Jobs

When I became Sir's slave I knew there would be a certain amount of visibility to our lifestyle, something that most people in master/slave relationships wouldn't have to deal with. Because of this I had to decide how I was going to deal with the issues of friends, family and jobs. The previous relationship I was in ended unpleasantly and resulted in my family graphically finding out that I was both gay and kinky. It was so different than what they expected and it wasn't something they could accept, so that and some problems have since taken care of that issue.

Friends were a different story. Before I decided to seek a master/slave relationship I kept my interests pretty much a secret. Since I relocated away from everyone I knew I didn't take much in the way of friendships with me. When living in Chicago with Sir I decided not to have to live with secrets any longer so I built most of my friendships within the leather and kink community. The few who were not, generally a result of places I've worked, were made aware of not only my lifestyle, but also my relationship very soon in the process of becoming friends. I wasn't ashamed and I wasn't going to keep it a secret.

I've been fortunate that the places in Chicago I've worked have all been Gay friendly, and the people I've worked closely with were people who took time to know me before they judged me. That's not to say everyone who knew me at work knew everything about me; information is always on a need to know basis. I always let them ask the questions but I didn't hold back any punches. If they asked if I was married I'd respond that I had a partner. If they asked anything else I let them know that I was Gay. If they asked what he did (or in some cases another discussion brought up a related issue) I'd say he was a writer and an instructor at a local college. If they asked what he taught I'd tell them. If they asked what he wrote I'd tell them.

People generally stopped asking questions (or discussed it among themselves) once they reached a limit of what they were comfortable knowing. In general they appeared curious; some were impressed or even envious that we could be so bold and creative in our relationship.

188

I suspect some were a bit jealous. They'd already taken time to get to know me so there was no need to panic about what they discovered. I don't recall anyone changing how they related to me based on what they found out. I never tried to convert anyone and certainly didn't try to put the make on anyone. We were colleagues and friends.

This all resulted in my being able to simply live my life they way I wanted. No secrets. I realize that not everyone can have this same kind of openness but I encourage you to find ways to move in that direction. Carrying a secret around all of the time does not make for a contented life. You don't have to tell everyone you are someone's slave, but part of friendship means that they accept you for who you are and you are betraying them by keeping such an important part of your life from them.

After Reading Activities

Let your darkest fears run wild by listing them in your journal. Then, just as you did for your fantasies, rate them as serious, easily overcome, or not really a fear. How can you learn to deal with the fears that have a negative effect on your search? Find an experienced player and ask how he or she would deal with the fear.

What things about your everyday life do you enjoy? Are they things that are compatible with a life as a slave? Have you included them in your bio or are they not that important? In any case, add them to your list of things to negotiate.

Reconsider your list of limits. Have you included anything about body modification, finances, or family obligations? Now's a good time to do so. Edit your list of limits accordingly.

Research what constitutes an abusive relationship. In your journal, summarize what you have found. See if you can discuss domestic violence at your next Leather gathering.

10

The Real Slave

*To serve is beautiful, but only if it is done
with joy and a whole heart and free mind.*[*]

Lawyer, housewife, regional director, salesman, marketing manager, designer, and editor are but a few career paths that actual slaves have — and at which they are successful. The myth of the slave as being weak or needing the care and supervision of a master is as far from the truth as one can get. In fact, the slaves I know who have been in long-term 24/7 relationships are talented, capable, and successful in both their chosen professions and in their service to their masters.

They are in a relationship of voluntary servitude because they choose to be, not as a last resort or a way to escape from life. In fact, research would easily show that the incompetent, the lazy, and those wishing for an escapist life are quite unsuited to the lifestyle described in these pages. I have consistently tried to make it obvious that the master/slave relationship is viable. The men and women I know who honor the title "slave" with their lives demonstrate daily the viability of voluntary servitude.

They have chosen to give a life of dedicated service and selflessness to their dominants, preferring their masters' wills to their own, empowering and supporting him or her in their endeavors, while still achieving success and recognition in their own right.

Will and Ego

Voluntary servitude is first and foremost a consensual act of one's will — namely the submission of one's will to the will of another. As

[*]   Buck, Pearl S., *Men and Women*, 1967.

such, it is simply believing, knowing, and acting in such a way that one recognizes and demonstrates that the master's will comes first in the life of the slave. His or her preferences, desires, commitments, and decisions take precedence over those of the slave, simply because the slave wills that the master be in charge, in control, and in command.

In many ways, it is most often a matter of priorities, since the will of the master doesn't necessarily negate the will of the slave. In fact, in most instances, both would arrive at the same conclusions, decide to do the same activities, and make the same decisions. When looked at as two complete lives, there are few times that differences of opinion really exist and when they do, it is most likely a matter of timing. After all, a decision to eat at a steakhouse one night doesn't mean that a seafood restaurant might not be acceptable on another night.

If there are major discrepancies in likes and dislikes between a master and slave, they will most likely be (and should have been) dealt with during the process of negotiation and may indicate that a M/s relationship probably won't work.

The surrender of one's will to another is not meant to imply that the slave no longer has a will, as he or she most assuredly does. Rather, it is that the slave's will is at the disposal, the service, of the master. The slave "wills" what the master desires. Likewise, it is not the abnegation or destruction of the ego that takes place, but rather the submission of the ego under that of the master; this allows the slave's ego be better equipped when expressing itself in actual living.

In practice then the surrendered slave is more alive, more real, and more him or herself exactly when he or she has submitted his or her will to their master. The real slave does what he or she wants precisely by obeying the will of the master, even if it necessitates actions that the slave, un-owned or without regard to the master's will, might have chosen to do otherwise.

As I wrote earlier, this willingness to do the master's will is a continuing decision, even if the continuance is, at times, unmentioned or unthought of. The slave is, after all, always free to choose to end the relationship and therefore, is just as free to choose to continue it. It is here that we see that which is called the "slave heart," as the submission of one's will to another, is a big part of the slave's expression of the real self, the one that calls and is "called" to serve.

Ego and Slavery

There are masters and slaves that take a more "Zen" approach to the M/s relationship, believing that the slave's ego must be nullified in some way. This attitude manifests itself in various ways, such as the titling of a slave as "it" or in the use of lower case letters when they refer to the slave. Some masters, for instance, insist that the slave only refer to himself (or more properly, "itself") in the third person, as in "May your slave use the restroom, Sir?" or "This slave requests permission to speak, Sir." I hope that it is obvious that I do not agree with this approach.

Conceivably, other reasons exist for the master to insist on alternative grammatical usage. So, the last paragraph might need to be read in that light, as it might be a legitimate practice. You know, I don't have all the answers.

Yes, the ego needs to be controlled and passions brought into line with the will of the master, but such actions are meant to bring the real slave self forward, to allow the slave to reach his or her highest potential. The ego is neither destroyed nor ignored, but rather is enrolled as part and parcel of what is offered in service to the master.

I fully grant that this slavish potential in no way eliminates the possibility of other "potentials." As noted at the start of this chapter, the lives of some of our subculture's most respected slaves demonstrate multiple successes — on one hand as slaves, and on the other as qualified men and women — living, demonstrating, and using their talents, both for their masters' and mistresses' benefit, and in the "vanilla" world at large.

The Basis for Surrender

Submission to another takes place in many ways. Much of that surrender is about specific actions and activities, such as the surrender that takes place when one is flogged or fisted. On the other hand, there are general techniques or, more precisely, attitudes, that aid one in surrendering one's will. Consideration of these ideas brings us back to the importance of knowing oneself. The primary basis and motivation for living as a slave is awareness of slavery as an existence in which one is meant to dwell.

No two people will express the sentiments in the last paragraph identically. Some see their slavery as a "calling," others feel strongly that they were "born to serve" or have a "slave heart." For still others, slavery is a path to joy, pleasure, contentment, or satisfaction. They know that they are happiest when enslaved, when they have someone to control or direct them, that a life of obedience is what fulfills them the most. It is a realization of something like the above, then, that is the primary basis for the surrendering of one's will. Without such a basis, there are no "techniques" that will bring a person to true surrender.

It is important to note a difference here. Though the idea of slavery is certainly very erotic to some, and sexual pleasure is often an important incentive in creating and maintaining a D/s relationship, there is more to this basis than just feelings, per se. If your motivation is only emotional, you run the risk that when the emotion passes, as it certainly will, there will remain little incentive for continuing in the relationship. For that reason, the use of the word feeling and how we actually feel must be considered in the wider framework of an inner knowing and a more permeating rightness.

The basis needs be more than just emotional, including an intellectual, physical, moral, and spiritual rightness. It brings not just an elation, but peace and a sense of security and well-being.

That said, then, it is the totality of experiences that brings one to the realization of the true slave-self. This totality teaches the slave to surrender; it must remain in the slave's mind as the reason, *par excellence,* for why submission occurs. Whatever reminds the slave that slavery is his or her path to self-realization and fulfillment is, therefore, the prime basis for continuing in such service.

Setting Priorities

Surrender, though, is more than an idea or an attitude in that it manifests itself in actions, varied by situation and the desires of the master. In general, though, it is safe to say that surrender is most often called for in the setting of the slave's priorities. One ought to re-read the paragraphs above concerning will with the understanding that conforming to your master's will means nothing less than having his or her priorities as your own. It is as simple as that.

The master may not be quick to set your schedule. He may not bother about domestic details or financial arrangements. She may never discuss the future, care about a calendar, or have a preference about certain things. Still, the slave strives to know the master so well that he or she is able to mirror his or her master's priorities. What counts to your lord or lady first, needs to always count most to you, as well.

Priority determines: "Precedence, especially established by order or importance or urgency." The master will, then, in many cases, set priorities for the slave. At other times, though, it is going to rest with the slave to estimate what the master wants first, even when two wishes present conflicting priorities. "Do I answer the phone or get the door?" This reflects only one of many conflicts the slave will have to resolve.

Here, the variations in styles of domination can be best seen, as some masters are much more controlling than others. Tasks that one might demand be done in a certain order may hold no such care for another master. What is important to one, such as starched and pressed shirts, may hold no sway over a master who barely notices what he wears.

Happily, over time, the attentive slave will learn the ins and outs of the master's thinking, and will naturally come to know what the master would want and when and how. This process takes time, of course, but is greatly facilitated by the slave's desire. Make your master's priorities your first priority and you will soon know what they are.

The Gift of Self

Though it isn't always seen as such, slavery is in fact a "gift" of oneself to the master. Seen in that light, we can reflect on the importance, even the sanctity, of that giving. It puts a different "spin" on what it is that we do, emphasizing the slave's high calling and negating the notion that slavery is merely an escape or only sexual in nature.[†]

The notion of a gift also reinforces that it is the master's responsibility to accept the gift. The master's acceptance of the slave's life into his own is no light matter and should never be trivialized as such. The wise master understands that the slave is a gift who keeps on giving, and therefore, needs care, control, and protection in order to both continue his or her giving and to have the support, encouragement, and satisfaction that empower the slave to continue it.

The Proud Slave

Society sends mixed signals about pride. Our country's prominent religions often preach about its dangers, while other institutions and citizens point out that pride in oneself and in one's accomplishments can be a healthy thing. In the context of self-image, it is important for the slave to have pride in his position, his service, and himself. A poor self-image makes it difficult to have a satisfying relationship, especially an M/s one.

The usual master is naturally dominant, aggressive, and imposing — traits that make him or her exactly what a slave is seeking in his or her partner. A lesser known dynamic is that slaves need the strength of self-image to withstand and complement the master's personality. The myth of the "weak" slave is not only erroneous, but dangerous. Successful slaves are regularly extremely competent, self-assured, with an inner strength that easily matches that of their master or mistress. Since mastery and slavery are complementary roles, how could it be otherwise?

Devotion

In all of this, the slave's personality is balanced by his or her devotion: "Ardent attachment or affection" to the master. Though we seldom discuss it and generally don't seek it in an applicant, devotion is built in the course of living the relationship. In time, it becomes an obvious attribute of the master/slave relationship. Happily, too, it is a mutual attachment

---

†   Not coincidentally, it can be said that the master, too, is a gift of self to the slave.

and affection, as many masters easily demonstrate their devotion to their slave, even if it is one of those little-noted characteristics.

The Last Word About Real Slavery

It is important to note that the traits of a real slave are not developed overnight. There is no quick and easy formula for becoming successful in your relationship, your service, and your kinky life. All of this, from searching to finding, from obedience to pleasure, are going to take time. As my grandmother, Rose, said, "Roma wasn't built in the once."

Be patient, then, with yourself and your prospective master. Let time inform your actions and your trust. Be quick to forgive and to ask for clarity. Be slow to discount your latest applicant as not good enough. Patience is necessary and remember that those who are seeking you will have lots of need for patience, as well.

Patrick Reflects: Being Real

When it came to this chapter I was at a loss about what to write. I've already written about being real in other reflections and some times you can beat a topic to death so that no one listens to it. So I'll take a break from the preaching. Instead, I'll give an excerpt from the journal I kept the first two years I was Sir's slave; that will give you some insight as to how I coped with things on a day to day basis and the kinds of thoughts that occupied my mind as I was adjusting to being a slave.

For me journaling was a way of communicating my thoughts and feelings to Sir. When I first became Sir's slave, my quiet nature and shyness, along with the fact that I was the fourth in the relationship (Master Lynn was Sir's master, Michael was Sir's lover, and Bobby was Master Lynn's live-in slave), made it difficult to talk freely to Sir. Sometimes it was difficult to be ready to talk when we could find time for it. At other times I was trying to sort out what were appropriate feelings for a slave; I was still learning what was appropriate and comfortable.

This excerpt, five months into the relationship, is typical of my thought processes as got to know Sir and adapt to my life as his slave. Hopefully you'll glean a sense from it about what real voluntary servitude is all about.

May 1996:

1st, Wednesday, PM — Sir stretched me out, arms straight above my head, legs tied together, and pulled the ropes taunt. Then he wrapped the ace bandage around my head, securely gagging me. Good thing, too, because the flogger hurts me, uncontrollably. I hate it.

I think I'm doing fairly well in handling the pain, though. I can handle it usually because it gives Sir pleasure. But on the upper back — I hate it. Maybe my back's just not seasoned, toughened, and needs time to become so. But I don't understand why Sir has to do it. I guess it's a pleasure I don't understand and don't want to understand. Perhaps it's because it causes me to lose control.

Usually I can control the pain, use it to drive me to pay closer attention to Sir's needs and pleasure him better. When it becomes extreme, though, all I can do is react. It hurts so much that I can't center on Sir. I don't like being unable to control it, not being able to overcome it, so it over comes me, and causes me to beg. And maybe that's where Sir gets his pleasure, from his being in total control, from making me genuinely beg.

But I don't understand it, and I don't like it. I even hesitated to put these words down lest it give Sir satisfaction and spur him to go to such extremes more often.

It confuses me as well because I can't sort out my place with this. I guess, as much as I want to give Sir pleasure, I don't want to give him that kind of pleasure. I do, and I suppose I should want to, and the fact that I don't want to confuses me.

For those few eternal moments I think I hate Sir. Maybe that's too strong. But I certainly don't adore him like I do at all other times. The odd thing is that I don't hold on to it. When the extreme pain is over I'm back where I love to be, to only want to give Sir pleasure, spurred on by the thought that he has finally stopped. Whatever it was that I felt is forgiven.

And I'm afraid to think that I might get used to this as well, because then what is the next step?

3rd, early Friday morning — "Go upstairs. Get a good night's sleep." It's 5:00 AM and I'm still awake. Maybe Sir doesn't realize that anytime he's home it's a good night's sleep. Even when I don't sleep much.

3rd, Friday, PM — Well, here goes. After sleeping on it some I think I can write about it. Or at least I have something to blame it on.

Sir scared me tonight. It was the first time Sir didn't seem to be present with what was going on. He didn't seem to be paying attention to what he was doing; he seemed distracted. He has a lot on his mind of late; Master Lynn's health, Sir's friend who passed away recently, and other things his mind has been distracted with in recent weeks.

Plus, he had to pay attention to Michael tonight as well. All of this seems to have made him less aware of what he was doing to me, and what I was able to take.

It started with the slaps to the face, something that always catches me off guard. The last blow didn't seem to have any control. It almost knocked me off my feet it was so hard. It took several minutes for me to be able to refocus and that's when I got scared.

It also made me start to second guess him and made me tense and unable to flow along with the play. So when he grabbed my balls I almost panicked thinking he wasn't going to remember that last night they were so tender. And when he beat my ass with the paddle... Everything he did seemed to go three steps beyond what I was able to handle.

There is a difference between being scared and afraid. I trust Sir too much to be afraid of him; he has played with me too responsibly in the past. We openly discuss things too much for me to become afraid of him. Fear is more senseless and comes, I think, when you can't control what is going on. There is no doubt in my mind that I would be able to communicate my need to stop, even if bound and gagged. Sir knows my reactions and body language too well. Being scared is something else.

Before he went to sleep we talked about it and he wasn't aware of any difference. Perhaps I was making too much of it.

5th, Sunday, PM — This is going to be difficult. I want to cum pretty badly. The paddle did it to me. I was rimming Sir and while he was sitting on my face he had the wooden paddle in one hand tapping my balls while he was stroking his cock with the other. Not hard taps, just constant and steady, the kind that usually makes me hard. But because I was already hard from the playing with me before I started rimming him, it made me want to cum. He played with my cock after that and I told him I was getting close to cumming. I thought he was going to have me cum, but no. He had me get off the bed and hold my arms out for a few minutes. That helped, because it put my mind on something else. It relieved the urgency, but didn't relieve the desire.

Tomorrow Sir will go out to Michael's which means I'm going to be tempted more. I guess I'll be holding my arms out a lot tomorrow night.

The other interesting thing from the weekend has to do with observation. Between the uncertainty of Master Lynn's hospital visit and Sir reading about the passing away of his friend it's been an emotional weekend for Sir. It's not a surprise, but Sir is as intense in his fear, sadness, and grief as he is in his happiness, passion, anger, and excitement. Often the fantasy top or master is painted to be without emotion; intense in his non-emotions, but emotionless. I'd rather have Sir.

6th, Monday, PM — I am amazed at how drowsy I am tonight. Maybe I over-did it on the antihistamines. I think I should switch back to the other kind; they worked better and didn't make me drowsy. Now I know why they cost more.

It's been a quiet evening; kind of dreary outside and that has subdued me inside. I worked until five because the "Quotable Quotes" had to get done. Then I went by to see Master Lynn. He's looking much, much better. His color is better and he obviously has more energy about him. He could also concentrate better. Everyone will be more at ease about his condition. I think I'll straighten up a bit and then I will call it a night. It's not often I go to bed early and it will be a nice change.

7th, Tuesday, PM — Sir is depriving me of his cock until I learn to beg for it properly. The dictionary says that 'to beg' means "to ask for as charity". Somehow that doesn't quite fit the situation. Sir doesn't seem to be interested in being charitable with Master Cock. The second definition says "to ask earnestly for" but that must not be what Sir is talking about either because I think I've been earnest.

The dictionary gives synonyms for beg as: beg, crave, beseech, (there's a good one for me to try tonight), entreat, importune. It goes on to say that "beg or crave applies to the act of asking for something one cannot claim as a right...", (which takes us to the heart of the matter),"...in a way that is earnest and humble and designed to stir pity." I'm not sure how predisposed to pity Sir is. He's more interested in his pleasure than in pitying me and it would be difficult to make a case that I need to be pitied. And besides, according to the definition given for earnest I think I have been a "serious" slave and I do understand the importance of Master Cock.

This all goes back to my statement to him earlier, honest and forthcoming though it was, that it is difficult to be serious about begging when I know that I'll get it in the end (no pun intended). Obviously that is not the case. I neglected the fact that the sadist in Sir can take a lot of pleasure in my pain. And he has done so, as is his right since I am his slave. As his slave I needn't think that I have any right to Master Cock, and should therefore be grateful when Sir is so generous as to let me worship it with my tongue and mouth or ass cheeks and ass lips.

Now to translate that into action and attitude.

(Note to my slave: I desire for your begging to include some or all of the following: supplication, praise, adoration, pleading, offering of self, request for actions that make me feel good [for example: please beat me for your pleasure Sir], thankfulness [sadly neglected, I feel], self degradation [I am not worthy to serve you, Sir], verbal self-abuse [I am not worthy to taste your cock, Sir] coupled with adjectives and nouns that describe my superior state [you, Sir, are worthy of all that is]. Re-read my column on "How to worship a cock.")

9th, Thursday, PM — The above note from Sir causes a bit of... apprehension, I guess.

I think I have been a good slave and Sir certainly affirms that in many ways. And to think I am falling short in such an important area is cause for me to be concerned. Why is it that this notion of begging for Sir's cock comes so hard to me when everything else has come so easily? The above note doesn't create anxiety so much as puzzlement. Sir has accomplished *making me very content as his slave. He is obviously worthy of such worship and adoration. And I don't think I'm unwilling to give it. It just doesn't come easily.*

I guess it has to come naturally, not forced or "play acting". Perhaps the key lies in the beginning of the last paragraph. Maybe I think I'm so worthy to be Sir's slave that I am above having to beg.

This will have to be thought about some.

11th, Saturday, AM — *I think it's time that I go back to my old way of doing this journal.*

I agree with Sir that too much reflection between writings doesn't improve it, only delays it. But dealing only with what I am currently feeling doesn't work well, either. I don't always have the opportunity to write when I have a "current feeling," and sometimes I'm too tired to have one. I'll go back to the old method, which I guess was a mixture of both. I always thought the entries were too long and rambling, but maybe that's my style.

Another slave applicant, David, is coming on Wednesday. I'm trying to remain neutral about that but he has colored the relationship by his distant behavior and rudeness. Something tells me that it's going to be a long two weeks.

As I say that, I realize that those are the feelings I developed from our initial exchange and the less than forthcoming manner in which he has communicated with either me or Sir. I simply dropped the matter as though I wasn't going to have to deal with David again and I haven't made any effort put them aside and allow things to start fresh. As I think about that last statement it also dawns on me that he hasn't made any effort either. If I were stepping into someone else's territory, so to speak, (though I know it's not my territory, it's Sir's, but I'm still here) I would want to know where I stand.

But with his imminent arrival I need to... (Added thought: I wonder if he has discussed the situation with Sir or if he has just ignored the subject of me completely? That would be quite telling)... but with his imminent arrival I need to let it all go, like I usually do, and not let it color my feelings. It's too simplistic to say that it's what Sir wants that counts, and my opinions and concerns have no bearing in the matter; that's unhealthy and foolish. But I know that I am capable of, both putting Sir's interests and wishes ahead of mine, AND letting bygones be bygones. Who knows, I might actually like the guy.

I do think that, for me, the more important issue is the respect he shows toward Sir. If he can have the proper attitude and can develop the proper frame of mind, that will go a long way towards how I feel. I suspect that my attitude and the high place in which I hold Sir has made the task more difficult, but we'll see.

With that dark spot purged from my thoughts it's time to move forward.

I am very glad that I finally have a permanent job. Not only was I concerned that Sir was having doubts, but I was as well. Usually, when I feel a particular job is right I am able to make it happen, and I was getting worried. I suspect that both previous employers had difficulties with the amount of fee that the agency wanted, but if they think a temp agency's price for me is steep, they would be shocked at the price they would have to pay Sir to own me!

11th, Saturday, PM — Being deprived of Sir's cock, perhaps is working. I hope so because I do miss it. Maybe that's not the right word. I hunger for it. I didn't realize how much until this afternoon. Oh, I have wanted to get my lips around it, and Sir has teased and let me get close to it, allowing me to get real close and mumble my words of worship, inadequate though they are. Close enough for it to feel my hot breath, and close enough for my lips to feel the warmth it generates, but not close enough to take into my mouth.

I have even occasionally chanced my ritual kiss before putting a condom on it and he has yet to forbid that. I guess because he knows that allowing it is almost worse than forbidding me to do it. It happens so fast, it's over before I have a chance to enjoy it.

But for the most part it has not been deprivation so much as acquiescing to Sir's control. He seems to know that I won't go for it without being permitted (though it might be worth the punishment — I wonder what would happen? Is it worth chancing the brush?). I am able to see it and get close to it. I am able to watch it shoot its cum, which is almost as satisfying as being able to suck it. That satisfaction comes not from thinking I am the cause of it, but more because it symbolizes the pleasure Sir gets from owning me and using me. It's a subtle difference, moving the emphasis away from me and placing it on what Sir feels. It leaves the control in Sir's hands; I don't control Sir, he allows himself the pleasure.

But I'm rambling again. I'm beginning to hunger for Sir's cock, and I didn't know how much until he allowed me to lick off the bits of hairs from where he touched up the shaving of his balls after I dried him off. He told me to lick it clean. I paused, not out of hesitation, but more from surprise at his letting me do it. I licked and lapped at it eagerly, in spite of the fact that I knew that all evening I would plagued with minute bits of ball hair inside my mouth. There is still one lodged behind an upper tooth, just long enough to be a distraction but too short to grasp.

I went at it eagerly and that's when I realized how much I wanted it. I was supposed to be cleaning it, not inhaling it. I forced myself to slow down and redirect my attention from wanting his cock to concentrating on licking the area clean like I was supposed to be doing, making sure it was ready for Sir's use of it later.

The "it" I refer to is his crotch. He used the word "it" but I understood that he wasn't giving me free reign of his cock. (Oh but that he would, could I control myself?) He wanted his crotch cleaned and I knew that meant his balls because the touch-up shaving didn't include his shaft, and that is where I centered my energies. I had just decided that I would end by risking one nice suck down his shaft (not for my pleasure, mind you, but to be sure it was clean and ready for later) when he pulled it away and finished drying off with the towel.

I hesitated too long.

Sometimes I'm too submissive for my own good.

Sometimes it's hell being such a good slave that I so readily put Sir's pleasure above my own.

Sometimes, maybe I shouldn't.

Sometimes maybe I won't.

As I was writing the above I remembered how nice it is (and would be) to have a long, leisurely suck on cock. Not active sex, at least for the cock, but just a long, quiet suck on a soft cock. Sir's cock, preferably (except Sir's cock wouldn't stay soft very long). He wouldn't have to be paying me much attention, he could be reading or working on the computer, even sleeping (trying to), or eating, for all I care. It would be a nice gift or reward.

But I don't guess it will happen anytime soon, since Sir gets such pleasure out of depriving me.

Sometime during the last few days, I have wanted to just sneak up and indulge myself. But I don't without his permission. I'm such a damn obedient slave..

Sunday, 5 AM — I woke up thinking I heard Sir call out to me and I sat up and looked over at the bed. It took a moment to realize he wasn't in it. Then I couldn't get back to sleep so I came upstairs to the computer, near him. Reading over last night's entry I realize that, yes, cock deprivation must be getting to me. I normally don't even think about disobeying, no less fantasize about it.

And yes, that hair is still lodged in the tooth. I think I'll go brush my teeth.

After Reading Activities

There are those who deceive themselves into thinking that slavery is for the weak, the inept, and those who are prone to failure. What in your life proves that you are strong, capable, and successful?

Some seeking to own a slave, seek those who are "worthless scum." What do you think of this and how would you respond to such an

202

opinion?

What is your self-image like? Does it need some work? What might you do to improve it? Is it strong enough to serve an aggressive, dominant, and demanding master? How do you know and what might you do to remove any negative self-feelings? Discuss these questions and answers with someone who might be of help.

11

Sexual Service

Now I know that success is Mr. Benson's cock,
however and whenever I can get it.
— Jamie in Mr. Benson[*]

Nowhere in the master/slave relationship is there as wide a variation in preferences and activities as there is when it comes to sexual service. Variations in gender, sexual orientation, erotic desire, health, and simple mores and customs cause a great number of actual differences among master/slave couples. Some M/s relationships, for instance, place a high value on sexual intimacy, with it being a strong, if not primary, purpose of the relationship. Others may desire that sex have a lesser, or even non-existent role, in their partnership. Although it seems that many masters are sadistic, not all are. Likewise, there are significant differences when it comes to preferred fetishes. Some may love ass-play, for example, while for others, it is a hard limit.

For those reasons, this chapter presents one of the greatest challenges in writing this book. How can an author cover all of the sexual activities and variations that we humans can contrive? I can't. What I can do is give a few general considerations and encourage you and your prospective partner to discuss the implications of your own sexual desires.

Fear of Intimacy

I have written, it seems, over and over again, about the need for the slave to surrender. This necessity is nowhere as evident as it in the area of sex. One would think that an author writing about sex in a book about BDSM slavery wouldn't take any time to discuss intimacy

---

[*]   Preston, John, *Mr. Benson*, Cleis Press, San Francisco, 2004.

but such should not be the case. As a matter of fact, it could be easily proven that intimacy is one of the least discussed, yet most important, topics in our D/s subculture.

Unfortunately, it's not discussed from lack of need, but rather, in my humble opinion, because so many of those involved in the "scene" either take it for granted, or use the scene for erotic behavior, without actually getting intimate. You may need a minute to think about that sentence, as something can be intimate without being erotic (the relationship between close Platonic friends) or erotic without being intimate (pornography). There are several definitions to the word intimate; the most appropriate for my discussion is: "Pertaining to or indicative of one's deepest nature; essential; innermost."

Intimacy infers that we are able to move past guilt, shame, and fear to open ourselves physically, emotionally, and psychologically to our partner. As a physical phenomena, it means that our partner has access to our bodies, their smells, tastes, sounds, and imperfections. All the prohibitions our parents taught us, such as nudity, defecation in another's sight, and behaviors that would be considered impolite in pubic, are commonplace when we are in private with our master or slave. I can still hear my mother say things like, "Don't touch that!" ....as I feel up my slave's asshole, genitals, or tits.

We probably expect physical intimacy. What is more difficult is to actually have it: to let our defenses down, to pour out our inner feelings, to admit to our fears, our prejudices, and even that which we loathe to someone who may use this information against us. Intimacy takes that risk — though to be honest, it is a risk taken with someone we have learned we can trust. Once again, we must return to the importance of earning and having trust, as well as the necessity of our being trustworthy. In fact, intimacy strengthens a relationship, especially one between master and slave.

In practice, physical intimacy is part and parcel of human intimacy in general. When we venture into sexual service, there is the problem that we too often think of it as being only physical; in actuality, it may involve emotional, intellectual, and spiritual intimacy, as well. Whether we expect it to be so or not, our relationships will naturally begin to include our whole lives. Therefore, it is always necessary to approach them holistically. To think "it's only sex" is to deny the important reality that all we do is interconnected, that we cannot divide one part of ourselves from any other part. Likewise, not all intimacy involves sexual activity. There is such a thing as a Platonic relationship, and as masters and slaves who enter into non-sexual relationships.

Each of us has been taught about the danger or impropriety of being intimate. Discovery and acceptance of a master or mistress is no reason to assume that intimacy will come naturally or automatically. It only comes over time, and in some circumstances, with a great deal of "work" to understand why we hesitate to bare our souls to the dominant we serve.

I would be remiss if I failed to note that not all master/slave relationships need or demand physical intimacy. Once again, our raging independence says that the degree of intimacy shared between master and slave is going to vary with all sorts of circumstances and personalities. What can be said, though, is that if a M/s relationship includes sexual service, there will come a time when intimacy will be desired. That's not to say that two people can't be sexual without being intimate, as they certainly can.

Sex can be as impersonal as a lunch at a fast food restaurant. Quality sex, on the other hand, takes time, care, and the opening of the self to the other as fully and as deeply as possible. Doing so does not come quickly or easily. We have to be willing and able to set aside our fears, doubts, and hang-ups in order to both fully embrace the other and allow a partner to do the same with us. Only by honest communication and serious introspection will this happen. When it does, though, the relationship can become the most valuable aspect of one's life.

Duty to Arouse the Master

In many respects, the master/slave relationship hinges on the will, desire, and explicit direction of the dominant. In the area of sex, though, there is one case where, with the master's consent, the slave can and probably should, take the lead. As Master Panman has written, "It is the duty of the slave to arouse the master."†

As usual, I will not make this a blanket statement; your master may, indeed, have different feelings on this subject and your relationship may be defined significantly differently. On the other hand, I can't think of anything better than for a slave to be attentive to the sexual needs of his or her master or mistress, and to exert every charm, trick, and technique to bring sexual pleasure to him or her. This duty is not to imply a sexual aggressiveness or the taking of control. Instead, it places a burden on the slave to know the master's physical and psychological touch points and use them for the master's pleasure and satisfaction.

There are two caveats to this "duty." The first is that every person is responsible for his or her own arousal and/or climax. Our genitals really do have a "mind of their own," and such being the case, it is irresponsible to think that someone else can actually exert control over

† I apologize to Master Panman that I couldn't find this reference in any copy of *Collars*, the excellent quarterly newsletter he used to publish, though I am sure that's where I read this quote.

individual, if and when conditions are such that arousal or climax is physically impossible.

I am not forgetting that slaves may be taught to cum on command, or that there is always the possibility of some kind of forced "milking" that would be effective. There will be nights, however, during the length of a long-term relationship, where illness, fatigue, or psychological concerns will make orgasm, for either of the partners, practically impossible.

Secondly, this duty to arouse does not negate other rules set by the master. My slave, Patrick, for instance, is forbidden to suck my cock without explicit permission; hence, he cannot resort to this technique whenever he wishes.

Knowing One Another

The best sex is between partners who know one another well, including the knowledge of their bodies and the body of one's partner. This knowledge takes time to learn. As beautiful as the human form is, it remains a mysterious and elusive part of our existence. Mutual exploration of one another is a serious prerequisite to a fulfilling sex life. This exploring needs be physical, as well as intellectual and sexual. Both partners, therefore, need to be willing to share themselves wholly and completely, in ways that are appropriate to the relationship.

Just as physical experience with one another is important, so too it is necessary to openly share your thoughts and feelings about sex with each other. As I've written more than once in these pages, communication is important if you are to have a successful master/slave relationship. That certainly is true when it comes to having good sex. The wise master will inquire about his slave's sexual satisfaction and the honest slave will be frank, forthright, and respectful about his or her needs, concerns, and fantasies.

Owning Our Bodies and Giving Them Away

The noun "property" can be most aptly applied to slaves when we consider sexual service. Giving one's body to the sexual pleasure of another is one of the more explicit expressions of surrender, which is at the heart of a slave's duty and commitment. In practice, of course, surrender as a sexual being is meant to be pleasurable to both parties. In any case, the slave needs to yield him or herself to be used for the master's sexual gratification. For many slaves, in fact, there is great pleasure to be discovered in the simple giving of pleasure.

This is easier said than done. The simple fact is that we live in a sex negative society; the prohibitions, beliefs, and emotional content of any kind of sexual act are often highly prejudiced by years of shame and guilt-producing teaching from family, church, state, and society.

208

Surrender in this case, then, means that the slave, when necessary, makes the master's sexual pleasure more important than the mores, customs, and ethics of his personal history. He or she ought to be at the master's service — unconditionally.

The "ought" in the last paragraph, as always, is determined by the master in negotiation with the slave. Hence, the slave has no conditions, though the master or mistress most certainly will limit sexual expression as he or she fits, especially recognizing appropriate guidelines concerning the maintenance of their mutual good health.

Nowhere will you see the dominant's priorities more clearly than in a sexual context. At all hours of the day and night (literally), and in every conceivable situation and location, the master may call upon his or her slave to satisfy his or her sexual urges. It is the master's right to do so. Here we see the need of the slave to put aside his own feelings and physical comfort to please his owner. In the area of sexual activity, the owner's pleasure reigns without qualification or modification, except as willed by the master.

This chapter's contents, of course, reflect my conceptual bias. Your master may, indeed, have needs that define different guidelines and approaches. Nevertheless, the slave pleasures the master with his or her body. During my interviews, it is not surprising that I have found no deviation, no matter the amount or kind of sexual activity, between master and slave, from this last statement.

Physical Intimacy

As I have repeatedly written, each master and slave will define their relationship in light of their own goals and desires. What follows reflects my own passion for sex and Patrick's desire for the same with me. None of this section is meant to imply that a sexual approach is the only approach, or that it is necessarily the best approach. It is, we think, best for us. What works for you (another plural use of the pronoun) is what needs to be done.

Though I am certainly writing from the master's point of view, it is simply fact that the slave needs to find satisfaction in the relationship and in the activities of the relationship, as well. A discontented slave is neither fun to be with, nor one who will remain in the relationship forever. Though slaves and masters may, most certainly, have different motivations, and may differ in what satisfies them, the satisfaction of both partners remains a necessary condition for a successful relationship — even a master/slave relationship. As Patrick points out, everything has its price.

I often start a sexual encounter with my slave, Patrick, by having him lie next to me on my bed to cuddle and talk. The prelude to what it is that we do, for him and me, is fairly tame as we quietly and intimately talk about the day, the news, the weather, or whatever might hit our fancy. From there, I stretch out my arm and signal for him to cozy up to me in a warm embrace. He is, as usual, naked. I most often have my shirt off but leave my pants and socks on, as it's his job to strip me when I'm ready. In the meantime, he nestles his head against my shoulder and often puts his leg atop mine so it is touching my crotch. I gently stroke his chest or head, perhaps caress his face, play with his tits, or stroke his beautiful cock.

I love touching him. I mean I *really* love touching him. There is an incredible variety to his flesh and each part of his body offers me a different sensation. His chest is usually shaven, though at times there is a feeling of stubble, if it's been a few days. His back is shaved less often, as it only gets done when he asks a friend or a visiting slave to shave it for him. Hair isn't usually a problem, though, as he is rather smooth and what hair he has is silky and short.

Patrick complains that I am too predictable in bed these days and I probably am. After nine years of playing together, he surely knows me well enough to know my habits, routines, and favorite moves, just as I know what turns him on and what he really only tolerates. He has learned to grin and bear it, though I hope that I can say that I have learned how to keep him happy, as well. My prick keeps him happy so it's not too long before I tire of cuddling and tell him to suck my dick. I'm much more adventuresome when I'm sexually aroused and I strongly believe that it is the duty of the slave to arouse the master. So, I tell him to suck — and he does.

In that we are compatible. Sucking my cock is his number one favorite thing and it ranks highest on my list, as well. As he scoots down the bed, I spread my legs and he feasts on "Master Cock." It is a grand position to be in. His face is in my crotch; his lips sink down my male shaft to kiss my pubic hairs and press his mouth against my pubic bone. His hands automatically reach up to brush my tits.

I adjust my legs on each side of his chest, feeling the warmth of his flesh against mine. I nuzzle my knees beneath him so that they squeeze his tits, as well. In a few minutes, I might break the action long enough to put tit clamps on him, as the cool of the metal and the warmth of his chest make a sensuous combination.

When we begin thusly, since I am flat on my back, his head, arms, and shoulders are most visible. It's here that I begin my first reverie into the beauty of flesh, as his shoulders are naturally smooth, his skin beautiful to touch. As I caress them, I feel the power of his muscles and the strength of his bones beneath my traveling hands. Flesh touches flesh. I knead his flesh and squeeze the muscles they shelter. I run my fingers down his arms, across the back of his neck, shoving his hungry, wet, warm, mouth deeper onto my prick. I'll probably begin to get verbal here, but that is material for another section.

If I were still in elementary school, I'd be diagnosed with Attention Deficit Disorder, as I don't stay on any one thing for very long, much to Patrick's consternation. So, in a few minutes, I stretch out my left arm, letting my hand reach over the side of the bed, and snap my fingers. It's his signal to get up and put his testicles into the palm of my hand, where I can touch them and take ownership of them, as is my slave-given right. It is a different kind of flesh here, thicker, and textured with creases. His testicles present a pleasurable feeling as well, as they float inside the sack, slipping as best they can from my fingers, but caught nonetheless in my grasp.

There are so many places on the human body to touch and such a wide variety of sensations to feel. It's not just fingers that touch either. My skin feels his, my dick enjoys his flesh, my tongue licks and tastes while my eyes behold and my nose catches his manly scents. Soon I release his scrotum and move my fingers to the smooth, forbidden skin between his scrotum and his anus. This is mine, as well, and I love touching him there, squeezing the flesh and feeling the ring I had put there so that I could control him. I slip a finger into the ring and stretch the skin. In time, I will move my fingers up to his anus, circling it with my finger tips.

Here is another sensation, preeminently smoother and, as my finger moves into the darkness of his asshole, I feel its moisture and its warmth. It is the power I have to break taboos that I enjoy. I can hear my mother say "Don't touch that. It's dirty," and I revel in the iconoclasm and the effrontery of it all. After all, as master I can do that with my property.

There will be more of this later. Now, his mouth sucks one of my tits, while his hand plays with the other. I feel myself, stroking my spit-covered prick. I move up on the bed, resting against pillows and the headboard and send him back between my legs. Now, I have the pleasurable view of his gorgeous ass. The two mounds of his flesh cheeks invite my eyes to view, and my brain to figure out, what comes next. It might be time for his tongue to please me.

There are few organs as multi-functional as one's mouth. We use them to eat, breathe, talk, kiss, lick, suck, bite, and signal pleasure (with a smile) and disgust (by sticking our tongues out at someone or something). Despite its wide variety of uses, I've yet to see a workshop on the proper use of mouth techniques in SM, though to be honest, it is mentioned occasionally as part of other presentations. My guess is that's because we have the unfortunate tendency to take sex out of our public teaching.

If you try giving or receiving a tongue bath, you will notice that it seldom gets completed. There is just something about a willing tongue licking one's flesh that eventually moves the top into a near-frenzied state of excitement, so that he or she moves on to more genital-oriented pleasure. Getting the full-Monty from a slave's tongue can be quite the ordeal <grin>, but then I admit that even if it's hard work, someone has to do it and I'm willing to be the victim.

After the preliminaries, such as talking, cuddling, relaxing, and getting naked, I'm liable to send the bottom to my feet. Even if you're not specifically into foot worship, it is an ideal place to start. Kneeling at the edge of the bed, the knowledgeable submissive takes one of the dom's feet in each hand and begins by worshipfully kissing the feet with small, tender touches of his or her lips.

In all of this, the better licker knows that he or she ought to be doing at least three things at once: using the lips and tongue to please, while the brain remembers that each hand should be lovingly stroking the top's body simultaneously. Did I mention that the best bottoms need to be able to do multiple tasks at the same time? Oh, we tops have so much to teach, though to be thorough, I have to admit that other bottoms can teach as well.

Polite discreet kisses give way to a nice slow licking, preferably starting at the sole of the foot. Now, I have to be emphatic here. The operative word in giving an excellent tongue bath is slooooooooow. In fact the top/master/dom/recipient will want to take care to teach the submissive to do it right, as he or she will have a tendency to want to rush the job so as to get his or her mouth on the genitals sooner rather than later.

Getting it right means that the tongue moves slowly across the foot and then the leg in a back and forth pattern, only gradually moving up the leg, being sure to clean every hair on the way. When the bottom reaches the groin, it's time to return to the other foot and then begin the tongue-climb again. Alternately, the master may instruct that the tongue continue up the torso, avoiding for now the genitals. I prefer the complete mouth-washing of both legs first, but each to his own.

Once the front of my legs are done, I roll over and have the other side of my legs tongued as well. When on my belly, I am careful to instruct the sub to linger at the back of each knee, as this is a very pleasant erogenous area. I especially like to tell them to do so. It's easy. Just say, "Kiss my ass."

There is a wonderful feeling when warm soft lips gently touch my ass cheeks. It is a smooth caress that is very erotic. Patrick stays there for a while, circling in to my asshole.

Now is an appropriate time for a good rimming of my anus. As an aside I will remind the subs that if the top needs some cleansing first, you may politely ask him if you can get a wet and soapy wash cloth for health and safety reasons. The good master will understand.

Next comes the expanse of my back, with special attention being paid to the neck, followed by a flip of the top. (Let them flip themselves, though — OK?) Now, the chest can get its tonguing, with an added emphasis on the arm pits and fingers. Which, of course, leaves the face to kiss, the ears to delight, and then it's probably back to the tits, since they can never get enough attention. By now, you'll see why the Old Guard didn't use Right Guard. The taste of deodorant isn't very sexy. So, if the master is hoping for a full tongue scene, he or she might want to forgo the spray or roll-on for a tongue-on. Conversely, they just might not give a damn about what the slave has to taste.

In all of this, let me remind you that there is more to a tongue bath than just a tongue. Continue to stroke and pet with those two submissive hands and, as you work your way up the body. Use other parts of your skin to touch the top's skin, so that by the time you're worshipping his neck and face, your legs are intertwined, and your body is touching your master's body.

And, as they say in France, "Voila." Finally, the sub can get his or her reward with a genital feast. The position of the face in the crotch brings us back to thoughts about flesh. I especially enjoy getting a blow job while sitting up a bit so I have a good view of the bottom's bottom. Now, I will instruct him to bring me a crop, buggy whip, or other implement of whipping and use it on his back, shoulders, and butt while he services my manhood.

I have found that the judicious application of pain on a cock-sucker or cunt-licker who is actively doing his or her job increases the intensity of the adoration and the fervency of sucking. For my money, those who don't actively link their BDSM with their sex, don't know what they're missing. OK, maybe they do, which is even a greater mystery to me. If I haven't shot my load by now, then I've obviously got more work to do. This, of course, is a great time to grab some lube and a condom and do some active fucking, Since the crop is already nearby, there's no time like the present to whip the slave's ass or back while ramming the hell out of his or her hole. Like I said, it's hard work but someone has to do it.

Affection

One of the more interesting and varied topics concerning sex has to do with affection. For the sake of simplicity, I'm going to discuss only the sexual aspect of affection. Tackling the "can a master love his slave?" debate can really get us off-track.

Simply stated, each of us, I believe, has an intrinsic need for affection. We need to be touched, stroked, cuddled, kissed, and held. This need varies from time to time and with the myriad good days and bad days we all live. Yes, I have cried on my slave's shoulder and I have held him when he's been depressed. After all, what we have is, first and foremost, a human relationship. Neither being a master nor a slave will change the fact that each of us is human — with all our faults, foibles, insecurities, idiosyncrasies, and self-doubts. Affection is a healthy antidote to much that ails us, not that it solves problems, but it surely helps us to grin and bear them.

Unfortunately, our society sends signals, especially to those who would consider themselves dominant, that to display affection is a sign of weakness. "Poppycock" is my response to such nonsense. We are human and being human means that we have real feelings that have a real impact on our lives. This is why slaves are such strong beings. They have to help their masters be strong when the world overwhelms them.

When, for instance, I was faced with the breakup of a seven-year relationship, it fell to Patrick to be supportive and comforting, until my sorrow passed and I could move on. Similarly when I was faced with elderly and ailing parents, he was there to console and advise me.

Yes, there is probably little doubt that the slave will be affectionate toward his master. On the other hand, the slave must acknowledge that the master's need for affection is not a sign of weakness, but rather proof of his or her honesty. Likewise, the master's or mistress' display of affection ought not to be seen as weakness, since it is actually a sign of strength. Besides, it can feel good to be affectionate and at the very least, it can be considered a reward or motivator for good service.

There are, of course, those stoics who won't allow themselves to express their real feelings and there are, naturally, those submissives who prefer that to be the case. Contradictory to this, though, is the fact that the masters I know are real people, who have the inner strength, to be free to be themselves, even when being so could be seen as a sign of weakness. Still, the display of affection is a very personal decision and I'm not about to pontificate as to how your relationship will be lived.

On the other hand, I think it's safe to write that the slave's display of affection is generally quite welcome. From my perspective, displays of affection by the slave reinforce all the best qualities in a submissive. Being affectionate says things like, "I am glad I am your property. It pleases me to serve you. Your pleasure is my pleasure." There is little that I like more than to feel my slave kiss me gently. Yes, I like my sex rough, but quite frankly, the tender moments speak more loudly, more clearly, and more deeply.

The Conundrum of Reversal

The title of this section is certainly misleading, as what I am discussing isn't actually a reversal. Still the newsgroups keep asking "Is it OK for the slave to fuck the master?" I want to laugh at the query. In my reality, the master can order the slave to do whatever he desires. On the (honest) other hand, even if getting plowed by a slave cock is the master's desire, it may not be the best idea in terms of maintaining the relationship.

That's why I use the word conundrum. We generally believe that the active (fucking) partner is the "top" and is in control. The slave isn't liable to be in the position of control when it comes to his actions toward his or her master. The idea of gender compounds this discussion, since women can "fuck" using dildoes and mistresses may certainly want to receive sexual gratification from the organs or toys of their submissives.

In fact, a slave who takes the top role in service to his or her master is still in the position of service and, therefore, there should be no problem. It is important here to see that attitude can express itself in many ways, even in ways that (erroneously) appear to indicate the opposite of what is meant. To put it another way, the dominant is merely using a part of their slave's body for their pleasure.

Life, though, isn't as simple as that. It would behoove the master who seeks such gratification to consider the ramifications of being on the receiving end in either vaginal or anal intercourse. Fucking, after all, is more than simply a physical act and has psychological implications, as well. There may be no problem here at all. On the other hand, the demanding master might be putting the slave in a serious psychological bind.

In fact, many slaves practically abhor the idea of being "top" in any fashion of the word. Though they most certainly want to please, there is the possibility that doing so may lessen the authority of the master in the eyes of the slave. Only the two in the relationship can answer this question. My advice, then, is to proceed cautiously.

Another piece of advice: The positions assumed during intercourse might well provide a mutually satisfying experience for both partners. That solution is for the master to sit on top of the slave and to use the slave's body to pleasure him or herself. Doing so in this position at least lessens, if not eliminates, the feeling of the slave as top and certainly emphasizes the fact that the master is in control.

Chastity

Another control issue has to do with chastity or, more correctly, abstinence. According to the dictionary, chastity is: "The state of quality of being chaste or pure." It should be noted, then, that one can certainly be chaste and still not abstain.

Many masters, myself included, enjoy exercising control over their slave(s) by forbidding the slave from having an orgasm. Slaves, too, often prefer this kind of control of their natural drives, as well. I have long forbidden my slave Patrick from "playing with himself" without permission. Additionally, when I play with his genitals, he is forbidden to have an orgasm, which increases the intensity of my actions, as well.

Abstinence over time is credited with causing the slave to increase his or her focus on the master, as increased desire for sexual release makes awareness of the master's rules, control, and presence even more apparent. The horny slave, quite frankly, is a more devoted slave.

There was a time in our relationship when I became concerned that there might be a physical danger in Patrick's long-term non-use of his sexual organs; so I gave him permission to cum whenever he wished. The net result was a slight increase in the number of orgasms he enjoyed. More significantly, though, I think that it had the added effect of making him feel less controlled and therefore less slavish. Although I can't pinpoint specific changes in our relationship, I think for the time of his "orgasmic" freedom, he felt and acted like less a slave.

Within several months, Patrick confided in me that he wished I would exercise more control. I re-instituted the no touch/no orgasm rule and our relationship increased in intensity.

The words "over time" in the above paragraph come with a significant caveat. It is important for the master to take care not to impose a rule of abstinence that is impossible for the slave to obey. It may behoove the master, therefore, to allow the slave to ask permission to cum and then to grant it, or to limit the slave's sexual release to a tolerable frequency. Obviously, this consideration is another one of those that is highly dependent upon the master's desires, the slave's abilities, and what they have negotiated.

For those wondering about the duration of abstinence, the longest running imposition that I know of is nine months (and still counting), during which time the male slave has had some five nocturnal emissions. I allow Patrick to have an orgasm about every three to four weeks, though there are times when I am more lenient and other times when I demand a longer "dry" spell, such as 40 or 50 days.

This topic raises the question of chastity devices. In my experience, I have found them to be fun in the very short-term, but generally unusable in the long-run, which in the experience of slaves that I have known, is only three or four days. Others I have heard can use such devices without a problem for weeks and months at a time, but I can't document that as fact.

When Sex Is a Duty and Other Considerations

The usual point of view concerning sex includes the strongly-held idea that the master's pleasure is paramount. Among the first things I teach a slave-applicant is that I want obedience, explaining that with obedience, I get all the pleasurable acts I desire. This thinking leads to two questions: "What is the slave's duty when it comes to sexual activities that the slave doesn't like?" and "What if a slave really likes a sexual act that the master hates?"

The first question is seems to be easily answered by the slave's need to obey. Unfortunately, it isn't always as simple an answer as that. For all the emphasis on obedience and surrender, which surely do influence the slave's willingness to do that which he or she might prefer to avoid, our relationships are still negotiated and therefore, do not violate one's prerogative to say, "No, Sir, please not that."

When such an event occurs, it is important to know why the limit exists. Seeking such answers means that together, the master and slave explore the feelings, fears, and expectations of both parties and try to arrive at a mutually acceptable resolution. In my experience, many limits are simply overcome only by the passage of time, which is an important element in the building of trust.

Another significant strategy is to mitigate the slave's reticence by understanding it and then developing ways to get around it. For instance, though anal intercourse is one of my favorite activities, there are times when Patrick politely, but clearly, asks me not to fuck him. Most of these occasions arise when he is tired or otherwise just not physically up to it. It's not that fucking isn't allowed; it is more that fucking now may not be appropriate.

Limits can also be expanded or removed by slow practice and a gentle approach. A slave's body needs to be educated to endure certain activities. An easy spanking for a new slave, as an example, may be all that he or she can accommodate. With practice, one is liable to find that tolerance builds and the slave learns techniques that reduce or remove the reticence.

On the other hand, there is much to be said for the slave's obligation to put the master's desires first. It is often the case that the slave will find pleasure in an otherwise non-pleasurable experience because of the realization that enduring gives pleasure to the master. This "grin and bear it" approach is actually much more prominent than we think. The act takes on its significance not because it is a sexual act, but that it is one of obedience. Obedience brings satisfaction and the ability to endure. Sometimes obedience even carries with it pleasure.

Masters need to ensure that the slave realizes benefits from the relationship as well. "All work and no play" does not make a happy slave. For that reason, masters ought to recognize their slaves' needs, either by rewarding them on occasion with activities which the slave enjoys or by seeing that they have time with others who will satisfy their libidos, as well.

Two examples will shed some light on this idea. First, though it isn't among my favorite things, I will reward Patrick with a good bondage scene once in a while, especially complete mummification. I don't find it difficult to do and I realize that it is a "special treat" for him. We are members of a local SM sex club, where we attend monthly play parties. This allows him the opportunity to play with men who will fulfill his sexual desires differently, and perhaps even better, than I would. At one party, a top tied him up and played with him for an extended time, using all sorts of sensory toys that I seldom think of using. It was all for Patrick's pleasure and there is nothing wrong with that.

If, for another instance, Patrick wished to be single-tailed (I think he doesn't), I would have to ask a whipping expert to do the job, since it is not part of my skill set. Each of these examples are ways to overcome limits and objections. Careful analysis of similar problems and an honest attempt at mutual satisfaction are required. Happily, they often provide solutions to either or both of these problems.

Another Conclusion

There is, of course, more to sex than just the physical activity we call sex. Rather than write a book within this book, I can only encourage you to learn about healthy, loving, and fulfilling sexual activities with your master or mistress. This process begins with the acknowledgment that we all have something to learn about our bodies and how to share them as freely, responsibly, and generously as possible.

In many ways, the gift of oneself, the gift of the slave to the master, certainly includes the gift of one's body. Learn to share the physical and sexual parts of yourself, and the lessons will enhance every fiber of your relationship.

Patrick Reflects: Sex, Chastity and Orgasms

In many ways, this has been the most difficult reflection to write, which I think is odd, because sex is so much a part of master/slave relationships that it should be easy to write about it. Now that all of my other essays are done, I can focus on the subject and hopefully, come up with something fresh and thought-provoking.

Though I readily admit that I haven't been intimate with enough different people to put this statement to the test, I believe that sex between a master and slave can be the most intimate, the most erotic, and the most intense sex there is; it can grow even more so as the bonds between them grow. I think it has to do with the higher degree of control, and the dominance and submission that distinguishes a master and slave relationship, the power exchange. In the vanilla relationships, I've observed there is always one person more dominant and controlling than the other, often not even noticed by the participants. But in a M/s relationship, those same behaviors are overtly consensual, celebrated and emphasized in a way that can give greater freedom to sexual expression. As I said in the reflection for chapter three, eroticism is the heart of whom we are as master and slave.

Sir suggested that I talk about arousal and the role a slave plays in arousing the master. It's a role I take seriously and the ways it occurs are numerous. Sir requires that I be naked when at home and few things are as arousing to a master or mistress than having his slave parade around nude, knowing that it's done on at their command for their pleasure, with every part of the body available. Arousal happens through affection, intimacy and obedience; even reluctant obedience can get a dominant excited. During bondage and SM play, the way a slave responds has a great deal to do with how arousal takes place. If you feel alone and hesitant and express fear or concern, it can dampen the sexual energy for both of you. Or you can put your head completely into it, embracing and encouraging it, and take arousal to new, never before experienced heights. The ability to arouse (or refuse to arouse) in a master/slave relationship gives the slave a great deal of control in the relationship. Use it wisely and carefully, and with great devotion.

Sir insists that it's a slave's duty to arouse one's master. I suspect that, even if you aren't consciously aware of it, this duty and power a slave has is the prime motivation for seeking out a master/slave relationship.

One part of sex that male wannabes, in particular, focus on (and slaves as well, I might add) is the idea of chastity. Almost without exception, they desire that chastity be enforced at the hands of their master, usually by one of the many long-term chastity devices on the market today, but the truth is, I've never come across one that will prevent orgasm if the wearer is determined, and I've never seen one that someone I know hasn't managed to get out of or managed to have an orgasm with it on. If there is one out there, I challenge whoever has it to try it on me! They might not be able to get back into it, which means the holder of the key will surely find out about it, but they can get out of it and defeat its purpose. As they say, necessity is the mother of invention, and determination runs a close second.

A serious slave striving for obedience and honesty with one's master won't try, of course, and chastity devices, at their best, do a great deal towards curbing the temptation that can overcome even a well-meaning slave.

Chastity devices do not intrigue Sir at all. He sees them as expensive, a lot of work and effort to put them on and take them off; they restrict his ability to have access to the slave's crotch (he loves cock and ball torture), and he believes that a slave should enforce his own chastity as part of obedience to one's master. Mind over matter, so to speak.

Others seem surprised by my ability to abstain (though they need to realize that, at times, it is very difficult and does have the tendency to make me irritable), but I think it stems from a determination to practice obedience. I take my slavery seriously and succumbing to temptation isn't an excuse. Below are some early excerpts from my journal on the subject.

MARCH 1996

7th, Thursday, AM — *It's only been 15 days! I was sure it had been longer, but I looked and the last time I was allowed to cum was on February 21 — the Wednesday before Sax (a slave-applicant) got here. I wanted to have an orgasm this morning and I fondled myself a bit at the thought, but I stopped; I know my will power. If I get it too interested I won't be able to contain myself. So far my obedience in this area is 100% and I haven't been punished in such a long time that I don't remember where it hurts the most and I don't want to have Sir remind me of that. So I'll move on to other thoughts. I'll just have to wait until Sir is interested in letting me have an orgasm. It's not been too bad, though. This is the first time I've really dwelled on the thought of it.*

9th, Saturday, PM — *It's 3 AM. Sir let me cum tonight. Yes, it was good. After coming back from the Eagle and after Sir's lover Michael went home we played a good while. Yes, it was good for me. Sir fucked me and beat me (not so badly tonight, or it didn't feel like it). And yes, it was good for me! Sir is downstairs sleeping and I will be going to bed as soon as I finish this. I'm one happy slave.*

I'm hoarse from the cough I've had and my voice is about gone, and I certainly don't have any energy left, but I am relaxed and contented. Not a bad trade-off.

24th, Sunday, PM — *I have been entering in my journal the dates that Sir allows me to cum so that I'll be able to remember, since I'm not allowed to do it very often. Sir said Michael thinks it's unfair for me to not be allowed to cum more regularly. Master Lynn's slave Bobby has expressed the same sentiments. While I appreciate their interest in* my well-being, my being is quite well, thank you! I was allowed to come last night and I did. Sir told me I had to cum in a rubber and save it for him. That's hard to do when you have a long foreskin AND a piercing. Getting enough friction to get off can be difficult. I doubt that he feels he needs proof that I really did cum, but I do wonder why I had to save it. I suspect I'll find out later on.

I have two thoughts on the matter of my cumming being controlled. The first has to do with the basic purpose of my being Sir's slave. I am not here simply so I can have a good orgasm regularly. I am here for Sir's pleasure, not my own. Not that I am undeserving of pleasure from time to time, but I shouldn't be focused on my pleasure; I should be focused on Sir's pleasure. I can honestly say that I am.

Orgasm control is Sir's way of keeping me focused. If I was allowed to cum when I wanted, my focus would shift to making that happen. It would lessen the intensity of the entire relationship, making it more relaxed and casual, because we both were frequently getting what we wanted when we wanted. It can be a double edged sword though, if I'm not careful. When you haven't cum in a while it's difficult to put it out of your mind.

This brings me to the second thought. I am still doing some thinking on it so my ideas might not be flawlessly formed, but this is the gist. Cumming is like an ending. Once a person cums, he's done. (Not Sir, though. Sir is so wondrously horny that when he has an orgasm, it's only an interlude; he'll be ready to go again in a few minutes (or nearly so.) You can rest and relax, and wallow in the good feelings it generates. But your attention is primarily on yourself. This is not criticism, it's just the way it is. A slave, though, is not done just because they've cum. In fact, it can be misery to cum in the middle of play and still have to be active and respond and obey until your master or mistress is spent.

I do enjoy having an orgasm, but I am also very content in being Sir's slave and giving him pleasure, first and foremost. I get great pleasure out of giving it. When we play in the evenings, or even when Sir calls to me during the day and has me stop what I am doing to spend some time worshipping his cock, it is a very satisfying experience for me, even when he is ready to stop. For me, it continues because I'm still on the edge, and it takes a while to come down from that. When I go up to bed or return to what I was doing, my mind is still on Sir. The pleasure I just gave him stays very much in my mind. Whatever is aroused in me stays aroused for a long time, and since I am fortunate to have so much time with so generous a Master, that arousal is constantly restored. Sure, the arousal increases as we play, and can be pure delight if it's allowed to peak to cumming, but then it's like all of the air is let out of the balloon and there is little left beyond the memory.

No, I certainly don't feel I am missing out. Instead of relaxing and *remembering, I can bask in the glow I get out of serving Sir and giving him pleasure long after someone else's memory has faded because I can still feel our time together.*

One last thought before I go to bed. Lately I noticed a different but related sensation occurring, especially after not being able cum for several days and the play has been rather intense and prolonged. It feels like it does when I have an orgasm and other than that I don't know how to describe it. It's kind of like the sexual tension is gone for a bit without springing the spring.

Maybe it's not more than that wonderful worn out feeling you get when you have exhausted yourself for a good cause and you just collapse until you regain a bit of your strength back. It's a good feeling, leaving me with a pleasant weak-in-the-knees sensation. It's intense without letting the dammed up energy of orgasm have its way. I'm still thinking this one through.

Chastity, with devices or not, is one of the ways we express our relationship, and there are always going to be those who don't understand and others who are envious of the practice. It comes down to the master's control and the slave's giving up of control. Believe me, it can be very erotic.

Sex between the master and slave might not occur in every master/ slave relationship, but even when it doesn't, it can be still be something that the master controls. A master who is not involved sexually with their slave might still control whom the slave has sex with, or when and how often the slave has sex, and even take away the privilege when they don't feel the slave deserves it. Our community is certainly made up of a wide range of people and practices and preferences. I'll never forget an ad I saw in one of our local community bar rags. Two lesbians placed an ad looking for a male slave. The relationship wouldn't include sex between the owners and their slave but they would permit the slave to be sexually active (with the unspoken thought being that they could deny it as well, which is part of the nature of master/slave relationships). The ad has stayed in my mind over the years because it occurred to me that it would take a very special man to be able to thrive in such a relationship (no, not me!) No offense meant to the women in our community, but you can be far more vicious than a man when you put your dominant energies to work.

After Reading Activities

During the interview process, it is not unlikely that your master-applicant will want to know your sexual history, just as you will want to know his or hers. Use your journal to write a biography of your sex life, answering such questions as:

222

- When did you first experience yourself as a sexual person?
- Who have been your sexual partners and in what kind of relationships, for how long, and why did the relationship end?
- What kind of sexual activity do you enjoy?
- When, where, and how did you learn about them and experience them?
- How often do you have an orgasm and how?
- What do you fantasize about when you masturbate?

Libido varies greatly from person to person. How do you describe yours? Have you ever experienced a time of heightened sexual need? How did you handle it? Have you ever abstained from sexual activity for an extended period? How long was the abstaining and why?

12

The Place of Kink

Variety is the spice of life.[*]

One could easily start this chapter with the note that the M/s relationship, as a subset of the Dominant/submissive relationship, is in itself kinky. After all, the acronym BDSM contains D and S. Still other kinks are found within this relationship; bondage, discipline, sadism, and masochism are often, to some degree or another, part and parcel of what masters and slaves do.

Once again, though, masters and slaves engage in these activities to varying degrees based on their negotiated relationship. For those nay-sayers, who posit that it's all up to the master's will, I will simply remind them of the "SM master" in Nebraska, who ended up in prison after his slave withdrew consent.[†]

You see, the kink in what we do is actually a slave-given right that the master can enjoy only as long as mutual consent remains. This is as good a time as any to remind you that I am writing about a consensual and mutually-negotiated relationship.

There are, nevertheless, numerous examples that demonstrate that slaves often submit to their masters' fetishes and that masters indulge their slaves' fetishes, as well. What is less known is that sadistic kink is not mandatory to the M/s relationship — even if non-SM masters and slaves are far out-numbered by those who enjoy SM.

In discussing SM with both masters and slaves, it becomes obvious that there are two kinds of slaves and two different ways that slaves submit to sadistic activity. It can be readily seen that some slaves are

---

[*] An old adage.

[†] See page 108.

masochists and surrender to the pain inflicted by their masters in order to experience the pleasure that they derive from it. What is less well-known, but seems to be eminently more prevalent, is that many slaves submit to pain because they derive pleasure not from the pain, but from the pleasure that it affords their sadistic masters.

There is, in the final analysis, little difference in the resulting activity but great difference in the why of the sadomasochism. There are several activities, such as cock and ball torture, face slapping, and using my favorite piece of plastic tubing to whip Patrick. Still, he endures my inflictions with acceptance and a sense of pleasure derived solely (well mostly solely) from the pleasure the activities afford me. In any case, the result is the same: I get what I want and he allows me to enjoy it.

We don't often consider that there are these two kinds of slaves, since the end result is the same. Yet, in practice, there are. For that reason, it is necessary to consider your own desire, or lack of the same, for sadomasochistic activity. Having done so, you can then either find a master who suits your needs or learn, as many do, to enjoy their enjoyment. Quite often, it is a matter of not knowing how to turn the pain into pleasure.

In practice, both the master and the slave will have to arrive at a mutually acceptable expression of their relationship. This isn't as difficult as one might fear. As a sadist, for example, I am content to inflict less pain on a slave who is less of a masochist, since the infliction of less pain still gives me more of a sense of satisfaction, since less pain, in this case, is more painful than more pain might be on a died-in-the-wool pain pig. In fact, for me, being sadistic with a slave who is not a masochist is both less work and more fun, since it is, after all, the reaction that I enjoy most.

Expressing Control

Sadistic activity is incorporated into the M/s relationship because the master desires it to be so or because the master wishes to "reward" the masochistic slave. It would seem that rationale is a given. What is less obvious is that there is often another reason for the infliction of pain. Doing so is a strong expression of the master's dominance and control. As that fictional fly on my dungeon wall would note: "Master Jack gives Patrick pain because he can." LIkewise, Patrick will accept the pain because he wants to please me.

Herein lies the source of many of the alternate titles one can give a slave: property, toy, pain pig, whipping boy, toilet, hole, bitch, trash, and someone meant to be used. In this context, the surrendered slave (OK, I know that's redundant) is there for the pleasure and amusement of the master. To the degree there are limits placed on the couple's SM, the master may appear less dominating and less controlling.

This is not meant to be a criticism. As I've written previously, some limits are both necessary and advantageous, lest the M/s relationship become injurious, illegal, or insane. No matter the extent of domination, there remains the need for the master to protect the slave, even to the extent of protecting the slave from himself and from his master.

As a complementary relationship, mastery and slavery create a polarity that affirms and intensifies the energy exchange between the partners. This dynamic could certainly be the topic of another book; so, suffice it to say that creating the flow of energy between master and slave is fundamental to what we do, even if we are unaware or ill-informed of what exactly transpires.

There are, of course, many ways that one shares energy. BDSM activity is an important expression of one's dominance and submission, of one's desire to possess and to be owned, and of the mystery of who we both are, even as it is an effective and enjoyable exchange of energy and power. The fetishes we enjoy give expression to inner realities and ought to be seen as such.

That said, one can conceive of a master/slave relationship that is, in many ways, less kinky. Though the term BDSM generally includes the concepts of dominance and submission, that's not to say that an M/s relationship can't be relatively "vanilla" and sexually quite traditional.

It is my opinion that kink is an incredibly wonderful way to express our D/s relationship. Others, though, certainly may disagree with me. It is, after all, their relationship that is being defined, not mine. As I hope I've made clear, the master/slave relationship is expressed in real activity between two real people. When the cock enters the cunt or the whip breaks the skin, we are talking about reality. Physical expression of our desires, our commitments, and (yes) our lusts lend a dimension to the M/s relationship that is inexpressible in any other way. Even so, I will try to discuss a partial listing of what it is that we *might* do.

I use the word "might" because, once again, there is the fact that you and your master will negotiate that which intimately, privately, and specially defines your relationship. What you two will share will be special: "Surpassing what is common or usual; exceptional." My literary skills cannot define what you will create, as it is your artistry not mine. The slave is the canvas for the master's unique creation, even as the slave creates a master of the most special reality. It is *par excellence* mutual artwork, even if the artistic creation is hidden from public view.

Bondage

The ropes, chains, cuffs, and related paraphernalia of a bondage scene express the control that the master has over his or her slave. As the slave surrenders to the bondage, he or she surrenders even the ability to move. The restraints say, "I am slave and have no right to move, except as you grant it to me." Bondage expresses the master's control. As such, it is one of the primary scene-related expressions of the relationship. It is no accident that the slave collar is used to express slavery. The collar is a form of bondage, especially in that is not easily removed and continually present.

There are, to be sure, many masters and slaves who enjoy bondage as a fetish. Others, like myself, use bondage as a means to an end. In my case, I use bondage to restrain my slave so that I can more easily and more freely take my sadistic pleasure. A bound slave offers two advantages: first he cannot escape from the pain of my whip, paddle, or crop; secondly he is protected because the restraints keep him from flailing about in such a way that he might be accidentally injured.

Bondage does carry one caveat, though a master who enjoys imposing bondage on his slave will no doubt see this caveat as not worth considering. In my humble opinion, long-term bondage, such as in a cell or cage, puts the master in the role of being a jailer, and a person who is a jailer is the servant of the prisoner. Here, of course, you will notice the laziness of my mastery. I am not about to bring my slave his meals, nor empty his bedpan, nor do any of the things necessary to keep him locked up for long period of times.

I also hold this belief because I am not willing to leave a bound slave unattended. Having written that, I will be quick to say that if and when I have multiple slaves, I will be quite content to incarcerate one of them for long periods, since the other slave can then be assigned the duty of jailer.

Sadism

Just as some masters relish bondage or sexual service, others enjoy sadistic activity. I have already noted above that slaves approach sadistic masters in one of two ways — either because they are masochists or because they receive pleasure in knowing their master is being pleasured, although that's not to say that a slave can't have both attitudes.

Though I cannot give definitive statistics, it is probably safe to say that many masters, though certainly not all, are sadists. Why this is so is not readily understandable, though one might turn around the equation and see the probability that a sadist would be attracted to mastery in order to have a ready and willing masochist on hand when desired.

My own experience tells me that I am a sadist, but the only reason I can attribute to being so is that it arouses me. I suspect the same can be said of masochism. We are who we are because it is pleasurable. I am not willing to venture into psychobabble or guessing as to the various childhood traumas that have made me who I am. Therefore, I posit that sadism and masochism are part of a master/slave relationship because of the pleasure they afford to the participants. If it's not pleasurable, avoid it. I would also encourage my readers to go back to page 178 and reflect on the evil of abuse.

If, then, there is sadomasochistic activity in your relationship, both master and slave will want to have learned the skills necessary to either inflict or endure pain in a healthy manner. Since *Becoming a Slave* is not a manual of technique, I will leave such discussions to other authors.[‡] I will remind you, though, that sadistic fetishes, such as whipping and spanking, like all the other fetishes, ought to be learned, not only from a book, but also from a competent instructor who both teaches and affords the learner practice and mentoring. Never undertake risky play without the knowledge necessary to mitigate the dangers.

Once again, I have to remind you that your search for a master ought not begin until you have learned the basics of BDSM.

Discipline As Fetish

Having written about punishment in chapter eight, it would seem redundant to now write about discipline — which includes spanking, whipping, beating, and other forms of what we generally call impact play (such as punching and slapping). I do want to remind you, though, that discipline is done for the mutual pleasure derived from the activity, while punishment is administered for atonement and correction.

I strongly believe that it is important to clearly delineate the purpose of the impact play so that the slave understands and experiences the difference in any given scene. For the master to contrive situations in order to justify his discipline as punishment is to sow seeds of confusion in the relationship. Likewise, for the slave to deliberately disobey in order to experience a good paddling is to risk destroying the fundamental relationship of trust. In fact, neither needs to create the opportunity for the sadistic or masochistic pleasure they desire, except to communicate such a desire to their partner.

If two people are not free to discuss needs, the relationship is in a dangerous state. For this reason, both master and slave-applicants need to establish the right to communicate freely early in their negotiations. If, in fact, the master (as is sometimes the case) will not allow such

‡ Suggested readings appear in Appendix D.

discussion to take place, then my strong suggestion is to find another master-applicant. Likewise, if the slave-applicant inhibits him- or herself in some misled deference to the dominant, then he creates the same difficulty.

It is fetish — defined as: "Something, such as material object or an often nonsexual part of the body, that arouses or gratifies sexual desire" — that is the primary characteristic of what it is that we do. In other words, it is fetish that distinguishes our master/slave relationship from the vast majority of other human relationships. In the master/slave relationship, then, it is advisable that both master and slave-applicants know how they feel about the various fetishes and that they discuss them in regards to their being part of the relationship.

In practice, you will find that the greatest part of the M/s relationship varies very little from the norm. Most of our time will be spent in the same mundane activities that concern the most vanilla, most average, and least "deviant" partners in our society. Once again, I will remind you that the successful M/s relationship involves a great deal of communication. This allows both partners to enter into it with eyes wide open, and a clear understanding of what will and won't be included in their lives as a couple.

Intensity and Edge Play

The sexual activity I have with Patrick is wonderful. With him, I'm able to experience intense emotional and physical states of pleasure. I don't want to sound like I'm bragging, but I think that it doesn't get any better than this. Not only is this enjoyable, I sense that it is remarkable. Why? Because we seem to have been able to increase our pleasure by safely increasing the intensity of our play and by getting closer to the edge in what we do.

Why do I say that? There are definite signs that point to deep mutual satisfaction: groans, moans, and sighs; exhaustion when it's over; multiple orgasms and orgasms without ejaculation. I experience profound relaxation and heightened ecstasy. Patrick and I routinely have sex twice a day and I think that means that we're doing something right! To say that sex at the age of 58 is better than sex at the age of 29 is a gross understatement. What makes it better?

For the sake of convenience, I'm going to write in the singular person, but be assured that what I write applies to both of the partners in the relationship. Not only do I get it "good," but my slave gets it "good," too.

From the beginning, we have tried to be honest with our feelings and open with our thoughts. Our years of being together have allowed us to get to know each other very well. That is very important, as knowledge begets trust, overcomes obstacles, finds solutions, fosters creativity, and helps us to be relaxed with, and understanding of, each other. I know what he likes. He knows my preferences as well. There is something to be said — in fact a lot to be said — for having a regular partner.

My feeling is that the sex is also better with Patrick because our lives are so closely intertwined. More time together actually translates into more quality time together. Not only do we have sex often, but we live with one another and do a great number of things together. Doing so is one of the things that has made sex with each other better. The first suggestion, then, is to improve sex by doing things together besides having sex.

The second improvement (but who's counting?) came when I discovered that Patrick likes verbal abuse. I used to tend to be a bit on the quiet side when it came to sexual play. Recently, though, I've made a concentrated effort to be vocal towards him and the effect has been pleasant for both of us. (More on this in the next section)

So, now I swear at Patrick as he sucks my cock and it turns both of us on. Patrick is consciously doing the same with me. Instead of swearing at me, though, he praises me, actually talking to me and to parts of my body in loving and laudatory ways. It's the opposite of what I do with Patrick, but the effect is the same!

The next attribute that comes to mind is intensity. We are not afraid to be intense. We can "let go" because we are secure with one another. I don't fear that I will turn my partner off and he feels the same way about me. So, the pleasurable result is that we have no (OK, few) inhibitions. Again, this doesn't apply only to sexual activity. We are free to talk about what we feel and free to do it, as well. There is neither fear of rejection nor fear of refusal between us.

From intensity, or maybe as part of it, flows concentration. Or is it the other way around? Sex is better when you focus yourself on giving pleasure to your partner or do the opposite and focus on receiving pleasure, depending on which partner you are in the relationship. So, Patrick abandons, or tries to, any thoughts about his own body and its feelings as he directs his full attention to pleasing me. I assume a dominant role so that I only think of my own pleasure and open myself to experience every bit of the joy that he creates in me. In one instance, he is fully active, while I am fully passive. Of course, this pattern switches when I exercise control to give myself pleasure, such as when I inflict pain or humiliate him.

That paragraph needs to be qualified. Each "part" of our sex play holds a different characteristic. I'm not always passive, not always active. When worshipping my cock, Patrick will be proactive, even zealous to please. When I change the course of the action, for example,

231

by whipping him, then he's liable to shift his attitude into one of complete acceptance and passivity. Likewise, I will, for instance, lie back and tell Patrick to make me feel good at one time, then grab a paddle and make myself feel good by beating the hell out of him. In either case, there is concentration, which leads to intensity.

The corollary to intensity, of course, is edge play: activity that carefully skirts the line between danger and enjoyment, such as breath control, blood sports, and extreme discipline. Skirting the edge requires significant trust in one another, as well as a deep knowledge of the edgy play. This is not a venue for those without experience.

Intensity and edge play raise important questions concerning responsibility and safety. For those reasons, competence is absolutely necessary. This is no place for guesswork or bravado. The master should not venture into areas of uncertainty or throw caution to the wind. Similarly, the slave cannot abandon his own safety simply to please the master. As written earlier, being responsible is the responsibility of both partners. You are, after all, both adults and need to act accordingly.

Responsibility requires that there be even more communication about the intensity of the edge play. Take time to reflect with one another about your fantasies and to "check in" with one another to be certain that the intensity is welcome and that edge is mutually acceptable. It is only by doing so regularly and honestly that the relationship will remain healthy.

If sex between us is great, it's because we share our feelings about it and are able to discuss it freely and openly. Though neither of us is lacking in the genitalia department, the fact of the matter is that our largest sex organs are our brains. No matter when, where, or with whom you have sex, use the head in your skull, not in your genitalia. Think, plan, praise, play, etc., but do so safely.

Humiliation

Here's a question from one of my readers: "What is the purpose of humiliation in BDSM? What is it supposed to achieve? I understand that some of it is quite a turn on, but I still don't understand why it is used. Is it supposed to hurt the submissive's feelings or is there another reason? This is a fantasy of my new dom friend and I do want to please him. However, I do not know what to expect or how I am expected to react. Can you shed some light on this for me please?"

My first reaction to this reader's question is that she ought to ask her dom friend. Many of her questions are best answered by him. I can't read his mind as to why he wants to play a certain way or what he expects in that play. Once again, here is a case where negotiation should take place so that both partners know what's going on to their individual satisfaction. Because of its potential for emotional hurt, humiliation, like interrogation, is only properly done under the right circumstances. Negotiation is a prerequisite for the "right" circumstances.

Humiliation is directly tied to self-image. If the end result of humiliation is a lessened self-image, then it most certainly ought not to be done. Our play is meant to please and empower. This is certainly one fetish where caution must be used, limits understood, and the possibility of emotional injury avoided.

Even from its definition, "to lower the pride or dignity of," we can see that to humiliate is on dangerous territory. Our play ought to raise the dignity of each player; so, to perform an action that may do the opposite raises questions and concerns. In answering these questions, I can only reflect on the very personal answer that comes from why I like humiliation. My reasons may not be the same as those of others as I see humiliation in terms of empowering, polarity and catharsis.

Some allergy shots work because they contain the substance to which the patient is allergic. In those cases, small doses of that to which you are allergic cause the body to build its defenses and hence disable the allergy's potential for harm. In the same way, humiliation can be seen as a dose that takes the sting out of the event, rendering whatever humiliates powerless to have its usual negative effect. By appropriating, for instance, a derogatory name to oneself we remove its power to inflict emotional injury. So, when I call myself a faggot, I take away the power of the word to do me wrong. By disempowering the word, I empower myself.

Catharsis is "a purifying or figurative cleansing or release of the emotions or of tension, especially through art; a technique used to relieve tension and anxiety by bringing repressed material to consciousness." This is probably the most usual positive attached to a negative fetish. Just as we go to theater and enjoy a tragic play, under the right circumstances, experiencing the negative humiliation can create a sense of release and cleansing.

There may also be the fact that enduring the humiliation gives one a sense of achievement, much like some people enjoy a good spanking or flogging because it "proves" them strong enough to take it.

Lastly, and building on the previous ideas, I have found that there is a great deal to be said about the polarities that we create in the power exchange. If, then, the power exchange includes the creation of opposites, might there not be something to be said for pushing these opposites further apart?

I came to this realization several years ago. I had been thinking about the elevation of the master, about the praise and worship that one might give to him or her. It then dawned on me that the opposite might be given to the slave, that degradation and humiliation might be the reciprocal forces. So, I have begun to look at my play as the creation of opposites and trying to discern if greater opposites create greater polarities and therefore, create more intense scenes.

Now, intensity can certainly be too much and one must take care that intensity does not harm. Yet intensity in play is something that we certainly desire and strive for, especially when we have partners able to reciprocate that intensity with us. Is it a matter that the lower you go, the higher I fly? Does the humiliation of the one elevate the other?

It certainly gives me a sense of power and control to be able to call Patrick a cocksucking slave, a slut whore, and a bitch. There is something in me that enjoys watching him crawl across the bedroom, lick my boots, or kiss my toilet seat in reverence.

Patrick has a very secure self-image and a self-confidence that is not easily shaken. Intellectually, he knows that there is nothing wrong with him being a cocksucking slave, just as he knows that he is not a slut whore or a bitch. He's also secure in knowing that he is the one who controls the effect those words or commands have on him; therefore, the polarities can take flight, creating really intense scenes. Hearing such words, or being ordered to do something humiliating or demeaning, creates a greater polarity and hence, a greater exchange of power.

Enjoyment is what it gives me, but is it supposed to hurt the Patrick's feelings? Not at all. It should affect him the same way that any other part of our play affects him: by giving him pleasure, a feeling of contentment — in other words, enjoyment. Humiliation, he says, is probably what gives him the most pleasure as we play, and that I never take it far enough. Thus the polarities have a lot of room in which to play out.

I'm sure more can be said if we only understood all that happens. In any case, I hope this stab at an answer helps.

Worship

If humiliation is a valid fetish in our lifestyle, then it seems that praise and adoration have their place as well. The slave's worship of the master is a little-discussed aspect of the relationship. In fact, it can be called the most secret aspect of the M/s relationship. Because of the religious controversy that certainly would accompany the acknowledgement of the master as god, we tend to hide the fact that such feelings often reside in the slave and to some extent, are encouraged by the master.

In the privacy of their bedroom or dungeon, there are some master/slave couples who illustrate this idea by their actions. I know, for example, one slave who routinely calls her master "Lord," another who pauses at meal time, bows her head and thanks her master for her meal. One master has taught his slave a litany, that includes such phrases as

"You are the lord of pain" and "You are the god of fuck." On command or spontaneously, the slave will worship the master with the phrases "I worship you. I adore you. I praise you."

For some, obviously this is idolatry, while for others it is a natural expression of their relationship. The best explanation I have for such activity is that it is consensual and, when present, often arrives both naturally and comfortably. Theologically, it is the recognition of the divine element residing in each person. The slave is worshipping the god in the other while the master accepts his own divinity. When this happens, the slave acknowledges his or her own divinity, as well, in effect saying, "You are god because you are human. I am human and therefore, I am god."

Whether or not you, as a couple, explore such a dynamic in the privacy of your relationship is your decision. Obviously, religious beliefs and taboos need to be understood and accepted or rejected according to your personal and mutual faith. Still, slaves have long been known to bow down to their masters and for millennia, masters have received such worship.

I can only say that such primal and essential activity is part and parcel of some, though certainly not all, master and slave relationships. This topic then is another addition to the list of things to discuss.

Care and Safety in All of This

Any rational power system has built-in regulators that control the flow and processing of energy. Hence, our bodies sweat in order to release excess heat; electric power plants have voltage regulators; cars have both accelerators and brakes, controlled by the driver who's paying attention, we hope, to the speed of the car. So, too, any good scene is going to require "built in" regulators that rely on various forms of feedback to regulate the flow of energy, in its many forms, between the participants.

The first type of feedback that we expect is vocal. That's why we use safe words,[§] such as "red" to stop or "yellow" to slow down or discuss what's going on. Vocal feedback, though, is really more entailed than that, as experienced players often acknowledge. The spoken word itself is also easily misread, as a bottom recently reminded me when she said, "Ouch isn't a safe word." The way one says "ouch," or any other word, is what matters most. Inflection is probably ninety percent of the oral

§   It is well-acknowledged that many experienced players in long-term relationships eventually forego the use of safe words, since their mutual ability to discern the effect of their play makes verbalization less necessary. Still, the slave never completely gives up the right to ensure his or her safety by asking the master to stop and the master should never become so irresponsible as to ignore clear signs of distress.

communications equation. For that reason, it behooves the top to listen carefully.

All feedback mechanisms, of course, depend upon a two-way approach. For that reason, good communication, in this case feedback that is understood and delivers the proper information, is everyone's responsibility. There is, after all, a subtle difference between, "Don't! Stop!" And, "Don't stop!"

But we soon learn to listen to more than mere sounds. Indeed, it is imperative that our eyes be constantly on guard for signals to proceed, stop, slow, or increase the activity and its intensity. Body language, really the most dependable gauge of the quality of the scene, remains important, even if it is, at times, hard to read. Tops have to be alert to signs of marking, abrasions, blistering, or blood. They have to watch for muscle tension, anxiety, and fatigue and deal with it appropriately. Bottoms, too, have to take care that the signals they send are appropriate. Too often, the idea that a bottom will "toughen it out" interferes with proper communication.

The third sense, that of touch, is only a little less important than the others thus far listed. For that reason, a good top will stop what he or she is doing and feel the bottom's body, especially the extremities. Feel for clamminess. How hot is the flesh and how sweaty? When you're this close, you can listen for, even feel, the bottom's rate of breathing, in order to determine that he or she is appropriately relaxed. This "touch break" is helpful too in keeping a good pace for the scene. The idea is to build intensity in gradually increasing waves, even to the point of taking a break and returning to the activity after a pause for a drink of water, a time to cuddle, or even (God forbid) a cigarette. These pauses don't have to be as long as the above suggests, but they do offer a great method to gain useful feedback. You'll find your bottom nuzzling and kissing and purring with delight, as you find yourself bringing him or her to even higher levels of intensity by using this gradual method.

The most difficult type of feedback to write about is intuition. Over the years, as one gains experience and learns to be attentive, you'll find that you will gain a sixth sense that tells you what to do and what to avoid. The problem that this method poses is that we too often miss this voice as it speaks so quietly from our subconscious. Most often, it's only the slightest of hints and our rational mind or our loudly shouting feelings overpower it and it is lost.

Good pacing helps us to listen more carefully to that voice, as does experience. Even the fact that we acknowledge the potential of our intuition to give us guidance seems to make it more discernible. The fact is that our intuition speaks loudest only when we are clear within ourselves, balanced and centered, and focused on what we are doing.

In practice, of course, feedback is none of the above alone, but a synergistic combination of some or all of the above between two players who are attuned to one another. In reality, this happens not only because they are experienced *per se*, but because they are experienced with each other. For that reason, first scenes tend to go more slowly and often miss the intensity that can only develop when true bonds of trust and understanding have grown between the players.

This takes time. Quickies can be fun and (mostly) everyone likes fresh meat and new toys, but the best SM is with a person with whom you've developed a long-term association or whose reputation is such that you're able to develop those bonds and that trust rather quickly.

A good deal of this feedback happens after the scene, as well. It is very helpful to take time, after the glow of the event is past, to share with each other how it felt, what was good about it, and what might be done differently the next time. Even after more than nine years of playing, I still check in with my slave, Patrick, from time to time, to make sure that my current level of intensity, my newest approach to kink, and today's favorite method of "training" are still appropriate.

Another aspect of good feedback occurs before the scene. Here I'm writing about negotiating what will happen, as this is a good time to understand what kind of feedback might occur and what is either expected or unwanted in the scene. It's interesting to note that in this part of the scene, experience may, in fact, be more of a detriment than we'd think; experienced players are liable to assume that because they have so much experience, there is little need to negotiate. I found myself in just that situation several years ago. I was playing with a person who had come to visit for a few days. The idea was that we would just explore what might happen as we got to know each other. We agreed to take things slowly and to leave our expectations somewhere else. It was a fine three days. I was on my good behavior and she responded really well. As questions arose, we asked and answered them easily. By the last night, things were going smoothly. It was only after she had returned home that I found out that she was disappointed that we hadn't had intercourse. For my part, I had wanted to do the same, but didn't think she would be willing. If only we had done our negotiations with a bit more attention to detail, this question could have been easily answered. Obviously, what I should have done was to have spent at least some time reviewing her stay with me — during her stay. I should have, for instance, used the morning after as a chance to reflect on the night before, and negotiating the hours to come. Oh well, live and learn. At least we agreed that there could always be another time.

As one of my readers brought to my attention, the discussion of negotiations is probably more properly found in an entry-level book on BDSM; however, I have found that we all need to be reminded of the fundamentals involved in safe, sane, and consensual kink. So, a bit of a refresher may not be all that inappropriate. Similarly, it's a sure bet that a large number of readers are as likely to have not had a good foundation in the basics, without which people can find themselves in situations that they later regret. Hence, this section.

The Last Word on Kink

Though you won't hear it said very often, it is important that both partners in the M/s relationship get the benefits that they seek in the relationship. If such is not the case, you can be sure that either the master or the slave will find a way to end it.

OK, I am forever reminding my slave, Patrick, that, "It's all about me." Still, the practical reality is that unless he feels valued, needed, and appreciated in the relationship, he won't stay in it. As slave, then, you need to be mindful of your needs and to be sure to both communicate them to your master and to find a master who understands that you, too, have needs. This is especially of concern regarding kink.

A good example is when it comes to bondage. As noted above, I am a lazy master and bondage is much more a means than an end for me. Still, I recognize that my slave enjoys a good bondage scene and therefore, take the time necessary, on occasion, to make sure he gets mummified, as an example, just for the fun of it.

Communicating the slave's needs to the master is often a difficult undertaking, since many slaves believe that slavery removes from them the ability to seek, and therefore ask for, their own satisfaction. I believe that such an opinion is not only erroneous, but detrimental to a healthy M/s relationship. As long as requests are respectful, obedient, and recognize the master's role as dominant and controlling, there is no reason that they can't be discussed. I strongly encourage masters to facilitate such dialogue on a regular basis. This will allow both partners to gain the benefits that first drew them to the relationship.

There is nothing wrong for a slave to politely ask his or her master for permission to discuss any topic that is of concern. Even when it comes to kink, good communication is a two-way street.

In all of these pages, I hope I have shown you that fun is a necessary ingredient in healthy SM, and that slaves have the right to expect that the relationship to which they commit themselves will be mutually satisfying. "Forewarned," as they say, "is forearmed." Be sure that your master-applicant and you are on the same wavelength when it comes to pleasure.

Patrick Reflects:
It's Not All Whips and Chains

I think most misconceptions concerning Master/slave relationships occur because people think that slavery is all about bondage restraints and play. That's why so many people confuse themselves into thinking that they want to be a slave. They love to be in bondage. They love it when they are being flogged. They'd love to do it all of the time; so, they'd willingly be a slave in order to have that much fun all of the time. Take a look at the personals of "slaves" wanting masters. Far more prominent are the desires and long lists of what kinky things they want done to them than pledges of obedience, devotion and service.

Some people might play out the master/slave lifestyle as a role or fantasy, but they leave it behind in the dungeon once the play is finished. While great fun, this is not real slavery; it's just acting, even if it's good acting.

Real voluntary servitude takes place all day long, from serving your master or mistress coffee in the morning, or in doing the dishes and laundry and cleaning, or in the preparation of dinner in the evening, and anything afterwards. The play in the dungeon and the sex are only a small part of one's life. We can incorporate it into a full day of service or even longer, with varying intensity but to do so takes a great deal of energy and at some point, you just have to come down off that high sexual mountain to experience a little bit of real life to keep you grounded.

But what fun it is! When you are a 24/7/365 slave and your master spreads your arms and legs wide and attaches them to chains and starts flogging you or playing with your tits or whatever, it isn't some negotiated scene that you've both arranged; it is a master having his way with his slave, using the slave in the way they want and how he wants, for as long as he wants, when he wants. For the slave, it's a time of pleasure and fulfillment, growth and new experiences, and downright joy. It isn't the focus of the relationship, but it certainly is a nice perk! There's a special energy that takes place when a master uses a slave this way, and it makes for some very erotic play that can't be matched by those who don't live a 24/7/365 master/slave lifestyle.

Of course, kink in a relationship must be a mutual interest to some degree. As mentioned in the sections on sadism, not all masters are turned on by sadism — or by control, or humiliation, or worship, or bondage, for that matter. It's no fun to play "alone," and if particular scenes are not enjoyable to some degree by both the master and the slave, it doesn't bode well for the energy of the relationship, and master/slave relationships are all about energy. Nothing is more frustrating to either a master or a slave than the inability of the other to accept the importance of a particular fetish, leaving that desire unfulfilled.

Just as unrealized desires of having a master or a slave will cause a profound emptiness, specific fetish desires left unquenched will cause a significant preoccupation and frustration. Therefore, it is the slave's responsibility to be open to serving the master's pleasure on whatever avenue it takes. Likewise, a slave with unrealized avenues of desire will find it increasingly difficult to serve with the devotion that began their slavery. Frustration supplants devotion in small, ever increasing amounts and it happens to both the master and the slave. This is why clear, open communication is mentioned so frequently in this book.

There is one last word Sir neglected to mention that is very important to acknowledge. Master/slave relationships are not always kinky relationships that involve bondage or SM or leather. There are many in consensual master/slave relationships where those activities just don't excite the participants. The power exchange and energy is there, as is the service and obedience and devotion, and the commitment of living this as a lifestyle 24/7/365 is just as pronounced. We are all cut from the same cloth, whether it be leather or denim or spandex or khaki, or even Versace and Brooks Brothers. It isn't the how of the relationship; it's the why.

After Reading Activities

Have you looked at the suggested questionnaire in Appendix B yet? Have you thought about your answers? If not, make notes for yourself about your likes and dislikes. Now you have something to talk about when you are asked about the topic by a master. Likewise, you can ask the master-applicant how he would respond to those questions.

Use your journal to express your feelings about control. Are you into bondage, pain, or mind fucks? What kind of control do you think you want? Do you feel you need it? Why or why not? What areas might pose the greatest challenge for your giving up of control? Are there some things that you won't let someone else control? What are they and how will you negotiate this with your master-applicant?

Write a letter or e-mail to a fictional master who has asked you about your sadomasochistic experiences. What have you experienced? When, where, and with whom? What do you think about pain? How does it make you feel? Note that thoughts and feelings are different. Try to explain whether you accept pain for the pleasure of the pain or for the pleasure of the master.

13

Polyamorous M/s

And David took more concubines and wives from
Jerusalem, after he came from Hebron; and more
sons and daughters were born to David.*

Monogamy and polyamory† are large enough topics that they rate
a book in themselves, as are many topics in this book. Nevertheless, it is
important to consider them as aspects of the master/slave relationship.
In doing so, there are several basic concepts that underlie the decision
that M/s couples make concerning multiple partners.

It behooves us to begin this discussion reflecting on the benefits of
polyamory, since we too often think that it's just a matter of heightened
lust:

> Ramey (1975) noted the following positive elements to polyamory:
> increased personal freedom; greater depth to social relationships;
> the potential for sexual exploration in a non-judgmental setting; a
> strengthening of spousal bonds; a sense of being desired; a feeling
> of belongingness; added companionship; increased self-awareness;
> intellectual variety; and the chance for new aspects of personality to
> emerge through relating to more people... polyamorous individuals
> tend to gain a lot of practice at communicating their needs and
> negotiating arrangements that are satisfactory to all... the beauty
> and happiness of a variety of forms of sexual sharing between

---

* *Old Testament*, 2 Samuel 5.13, Revised Standard Version.

† A more detailed discussion about polyamory can be found in *Polyamory, The New*
Love Without Limits by Dr. Deborah Anapol, IntiNet Resource Center, San Raphael, CA,
1997.

consenting adults are affirmed.[‡]

In fact, the question of multiple partners is often the first "make or break" point in the negotiations between master and slave-applicants. Many slave-applicants are searching for a monogamous relationship, while many masters, not surprisingly, want to reserve the right to own multiple slaves. Nevertheless, there is no general consensus on this issue. More than once, I have been rejected as the possible master of a slave-applicant because I reserve the right to have sex with whomever I choose, while I have found many slave-applicants who hope to be used by more than one top.

There are monogamous couples; couples who allow both parties to enjoy other partners, who may or may not be intimate with the third partner; masters who allow their slaves to serve others, though usually only with permission; and masters who live by the double standard that they can have other partners, while their slaves serve only them.

The word polyamory refers to the concept of "many lovers," though it is generally applied to any committed relationship that is open to the addition of others as sexual partners. In fact, how it is open varies greatly among polyamorous couples. In researching alternative relationships, I have come to the conclusion that they seem to fall into three categories: monogamous, familial, and promiscuous.

Monogamy

In my years of struggle with the question of plurality in relationships, I've come to the conclusion that some people are naturally monogamous, while for others, such a lifestyle is highly improbable, if not impossible. In the master/slave dynamic, it is not uncommon for there to be a commitment to monogamy, especially between married couples, though it is also found between gay and lesbian couples, as well.

On the other hand, we may take monogamy as a given much too quickly, since it is certainly seen as the norm in sexual relationships. There is overwhelming social pressure to enter into a monogamous relationship, even if it isn't marriage and few seem to even think that polyamory is possible, much less right or enjoyable.

As long as infidelity is not a problem for either partner, monogamy certainly offers the easiest dynamic, as there is only one relationship that needs to be kept healthy. Compounding relationships with multiple partners is an exponential affair and having multiple partners quickly makes communication, support, trust, and love more difficult.

‡ Weitzman, Geri D., *What Psychology Professionals Should Know About Polyamory*, 8th Annual Diversity Conference, Albany, NY, 1999.

The question of being monogamous or not, then, often depends upon the personality of the partners and should be addressed early in the negotiation process. As a matter of fact, it is often one of the earliest deciding factors in ascertaining the suitability of a prospect. Either you agree that you are seeking the same degree and kind of openness in your partnership or you're not going to be compatible. This issue, in fact, is often so important that it is one of the criteria listed in the applicant's personal ad. Doing so is a good idea, since it saves both parties the time otherwise wasted when they have divergent views on the issue.

On the other hand, the issue of monogamy often hinges on one's knowledge of self. Too often, applicants underestimate their need for monogamy or for plural partners, being willing to compromise that which they might prefer for the satisfaction of the present relationship. I believe that, in general, such an approach only postpones an inevitable conflict. In time, the monogamous partner will want monogamy or the more promiscuous partner will want extra-partnership sex, thereby causing the possibility of a serious conflict. I grant that many couples, when faced with such a clash, find ways to resolve it, but I favor prevention over cure in this regard.

Whether you are a one-man man or woman, or a one-woman woman or man, ought to be recognized and negotiated before trouble brews through jealousy or faithlessness. It is also important to note that mastery does not give the master the right to unilaterally abrogate the agreement to be monogamous. That is not to say that the relationship can't be redefined at some time, as it most certainly can be, but doing so must consider the needs and expectations of both parties. Reforming an open relationship to a monogamous one requires the same standard of agreement, as well.

Polyamory

The second kind of relationship is one which is open to multiple partners who, in fact, mutually share in the relationship. This, then, means that all the individuals involved have a relationship of *some kind* with every other member. I write this in order to distinguish a polyamorous relationship from one that is only open. Too often, open relationships are thought to be polyamorous when such is not the case.

The participants in a polyamorous relationship will have some kind commitment, friendship, knowledge, and trust of and with all the other members. In practice, this means that there is usually some formal introduction of the person joining the relationship, followed by a time of trial belonging, and eventual acceptance by all parties of the newest member. In highly structured relationships, this acceptance is rather formal. In other poly relationships, it will obviously be more relaxed.

Openness may, in fact, be part of a polyamorous relationship, in that the partners — and here it is most prevalent that it is the master who is playing around — allow for promiscuity, with the understanding that such activity is sanctioned as a means of eventually adding new members to the relationship. Other polyamorous relationships might require that any prospective member become socially acquainted with all the partners before the intimacy of sex is added to the mix. In this situation, you might see, for instance, a personal ad that reads, in part, "Master and slave seek second slave," or "Two masters seek slave to serve them."

In any case, the addition of another person into a relationship requires the assent of all parties in the relationship. This may seem counter-intuitive, as one might assume that the master will get his or her way and that the slave won't have much to say about who is or isn't included. Interviews with viable master/slave couples prove otherwise, as slaves are often consulted, listened to, and regarded as valuable confidants and advisors to their masters. This, of course, is logical, as both parties, master or slave, have a significant investment in the nurturing, protection, and growth of their M/s relationship.

In the final analysis, I will certainly grant that the master will have the final word on including new members into the group. In practice, though, a master who ignores the counsel of a trusted submissive may well be inviting disaster. Obviously, here is a situation where early understanding of the nature and practice of polyamory can make or break a relationship. The reality is that the wise master understands and respects the value of the present relationship and therefore, will not jeopardize it by bringing in another participant to the detriment of the first slave's feelings, security, and happiness.

Promiscuity

The third option is promiscuity, a name I am giving to what we generally call "open relationships." Here, one or both of the partners are free to have sexual relationships with whomever they choose and who they choose is of little or no concern to the other partner. Often, the one with whom they are having the encounter is unknown to the other partner. This arrangement also has it own set of rules. Some couples keep their extra-relational affairs hidden, others just don't tell details, others do it at agreed upon times or in agreed upon places.

I once had a lover who I encouraged to meet other men and to enjoy them sexually, though I never participated in his outside relationships and he preferred not to be part of mine.

I arrange a tryst whenever I have the hankering, the time, and a willing partner. My slave, Patrick, would have to get my permission first, except when at the clubhouse, where he is free to play with whomever asks him. This rule, of course, is based on the fact that "I share my toys" with my brother Leather men. Similarly, others may have the same kind of rule when attending parties, conventions, or in a public play space.

It is more common for the master to be the promiscuous one in the relationship, though some masters, recognizing the sexual needs of their slaves, allow them to enjoy extra-relational sexual activities, as well. This model is one under which I lived when I was Master Lynn's slave.

Infidelity

To write about being faithful in a book about alternative relationships seems to be an oxymoron, but in reality such is not the case. Any relationship built on trust, as the master/slave relationship certainly is, must recognize the need to be faithful. What is divergent from the usual discussion of fidelity[§] is that we are not considering faithfulness to an external directive, such as church doctrine or societal expectations but rather to an agreed upon standard recognized as the "rule" for the couple making the agreement.

Fidelity is faithfulness to the commitments of the agreement, rather than to some third party expectation. Once again we see the importance of discussion, expectations, and mutual agreement. Whether a relationship will be monogamous, polyamorous, and promiscuous must be addressed and clearly understood by both parties.

The Need for Knowledge of Self

There are few areas in the M/s relationship where it is more important to know what you want and what you can handle than when considering extra-relational sex. As stated above, it is not uncommon for people to mitigate their true feelings about an open relationship, to try to convince themselves and their prospective partner, that the relationship under consideration is viable. In fact, almost any relationship is going to be viable in the short-run; therefore, doing so doesn't create a problem until the relationship enters the long-term stage.

It is best to honestly understand your own feelings and need in this regard and to effectively communicate them to your applicant. Thinking that you can overcome differences of opinion at a later date, or that you will be able to convince your partner (after the commitment is made) to change the relationship, is to enter difficult territory. In practice, it is best to agree upon the kind of relationship you will have long before

§   For a fuller discussion of ethics in BDSM relationships, see *The Ethical Slut, a Guide to Infinite Sexual Possibilities*, by Dossie Easton and Catherine A. Liszt, Greenery Press, Emeryville, CA, 1997.

you both become so emotionally, fiscally, and intellectually committed to one another that ending the negotiations becomes traumatic.

Here, the rule about not being able to change your partner is very important. Too often, it seems, couples enter into committed relationships harboring the idea that they will eventually change a partner's stance on a given topic. For better or for worse, that seldom happens.

My first lover and I failed to discuss our long-term expectations about having an open relationship. I entered into the partnership with the expectation that we would start out monogamously, but we would probably open up the relationship over time, allowing each of us to play around. My lover expected that over time, we would become more closely committed, so that there would be no thought of being sexually open. We both expected changes; unfortunately, we expected changes that led to opposing behaviors. These silent discrepancies in our relationship views ultimately caused the end of our partnership.

That's not to say that each person can't or won't change, as each certainly will. Likewise, relationships naturally evolve over time, as well. The caveat arises when the expectation is of a certain kind of change, especially in something as fundamental as sexual activity. The solution, then, is to know what you want, find out what your prospective partner wants, and confirm that you are compatible and comfortable with whatever arrangements you mutually agree upon. To neglect or postpone this agreement will pave a path to the probability of eventual disagreement.

Three-Ways and More

For those couples who agree upon some kind of open relationship, one of the options is that sexual activity at times include a third (or more) person. Popularly called "three-ways," they offer potentially exciting, as well as risky, activity. In non-monogamous relationships, three-ways offer both variety and a way to express the master/slave dynamic. There are many ways to illustrate the possibilities, such as one master with two slaves, two masters and one slave, and the master-slave-boy triad.

For masters, two slaves offer double pleasure, not to mention an opportunity for voyeurism: enjoying two slaves at play. Problems arise in this scenario when one of the slaves is bored with the activity, when the slaves do not enjoy one another, or when one slave is forced to adopt a "top" mode over the other. On the other hand, three-ways can offer a topping option to a slave who wishes to do so, provides a venue for slaves to "entertain" the master, and can, in fact, be exciting for all involved.

Similarly, two masters might find enjoyment in sharing a slave.

Scenarios such as this are common as well, especially if two masters have a strong attraction to each other or if the slave has a high level of sexual need. It also provides an excellent opportunity for a more experienced master to mentor a less experienced one.

Note that having an open relationship does not necessitate having three-ways. In fact most couples in an open relationship do not usually include a third party in their sexual activity.

Jealousy

The primary obstacle to pursuing multiple relationships, especially when it involves sexual ones, is the very real possibility that one or both of the partners will become jealous: "Fearful or wary of being supplanted, especially apprehensive of the loss of another's affection." Questions about jealously, in fact, are prevalent whenever discussions turn to any of the varieties of multiple partnerships.

For this reason, it is imperative that any applicants or partners considering opening a relationship to others must evaluate how secure each of them is with both the concept of openness, and with the strength of their partnership. Experience shows that it takes confident and self-assured partners to successfully navigate the waters of polyamorous or open relationships. If either partner experiences self-doubt or a lack of confidence in the health and permanence of the relationship, it's probably a sure sign that adding another, in whatever fashion is chosen, is not going to bring any real benefit to the primary relationship.

Too often, partners resort to open relationships as a conduit to solving problems in their relationship. Sadly, doing so often causes further deterioration in the primary relationship — much like having another child in order to "save the marriage" only postpones the divorce.

It is imperative that couples wishing to experience multiple partners, then, come to terms about the security each of them enjoys in the relationship. Note that jealously is primarily a fear and therefore, must be dealt with honestly and directly, as such. That is not to say that simply dismissing jealous feelings as fear will solve the problem. Instead, conscious efforts must be made by all parties to assure that all concerned understand the psychological needs that they have for security, acceptance, and the permanence of the relationship.

I cannot emphasize this too strongly. The decision to attempt anything beyond a monogamous relationship must not be made lightly. The partners must not only affirm their commitment to each other, but also share a deep sense of security with one another. It is important to understand that even a strong sense of security can be easily eroded when there is talk of opening a relationship. For that reason, the subject, especially between partners, needs to be broached carefully and lovingly.

Those in an open relationship must recognize that both partners are valued members of the relationship and that neither can approach the other from a position of powerlessness, fear, or self-doubt. In fact, only a strong and self-confident individual can freely allow his or her partner to attempt extra-relationship play.

Wishing to maintain a monogamous relationship, on the other hand, must not be seen as a sign of weakness. None of the options offered in this chapter is superior to any other. Rather, the ideal option will always be the one which best conforms to the needs, desires, and continuing growth of the individual. If you cannot create such a relationship with your current applicant, that is a sure sign to move on in order to find one who seeks the same kind of relationship as you.

Families and Stables

You will find a significant number of kinky folk who espouse the idea of Leather family. Masters also use the term "stable" for a familial type of arrangement that includes multiple slaves and, as often as not, more than one dominant. In practice, you will find a healthy subset of lifestylers who enjoy such multiplicity, though frankly, the statistics show that the idea of close family is rarer than the popularity of the topic would indicate.

The idea of Leather family, it should be noted, does not, in itself, exclude monogamous couples; whether the idea of family includes sexual activity is certainly a consideration that can easily vary from couple to couple and family to family. Very often, in fact, families include individuals who have never had sex with any of the others and where there is no expectation of sex ever occurring.

In practice, most family-labeled relationships include multiple participants, with the reality that few actually live together, and there is much less sexual interaction between "family" members than one would expect. This is not to downplay the importance of interpersonal and intimate relationships among them. To the contrary, many small families live quite well, just not according to what seem to be general expectations.

A typical BDSM family would include a core group, {ADD THIS PHRASE??? the Leather equivalent of a nuclear family,} such as a master and his or her slave(s); with part-time participants in their social and sexual life; and others who are considered "family," by reason of close friendship, actual interdependencies, and mutual support and enjoyment. The non-core family members do not live with the core, but are generally involved for some of their social life, in time of emergency or need, and for special occasions such as holidays, family celebrations, and other types of visitations. Many of these people may have previously been more closely involved in the life of family but have since scaled back their participation for reasons of career, distance, or the natural change in inclination, intimate relationships, or other pressing needs.

At present (Late 2004) our family consists of myself and Patrick, Master Lynn who lives in a northern suburb and spends an occasional weekend or evening with us, Matt who has just signed a six month slave contract and who visits on most weekends, Joel who lives in Philadelphia and visits for two or three weekends a year, mostly around holidays, David a young master here in the city whom we have mentored since his coming into leather some seven years ago, Donna, a long-standing friend of mine from San Antonio, and Elaine, a women who lives in San Diego and keeps in touch, primarily with Patrick, by phone and visits yearly. Added to that core are several very close friends and many other friends who mean much to some or all us.

Alpha and Beta Slaves

It's rather popular these days for masters and slaves to consider one slave (in a household with multiple submissives) to be the alpha slave, while the others have a lower place in the family pecking order. This alpha slave may have dominant tendencies or may be a more senior partner with the master — either in age, duration of their relationship, or experience.

As Master Lynn's slave, for instance, I often dominated his other slave Bobby and was seen in an alpha role to him. This relationship reflected both the fact that I had been Master Lynn's slave before he had collared Bobby, and that I was generally dominant in most of my other relationships, as well. In fact, I introduced Bobby to Master Lynn when Bobby had come to Chicago to interview me for the position of being my slave.

In any case, when there are multiple partners in a relationship, there will naturally arise some kind of "pecking order." To think otherwise is to deny fundamental characteristics of human living. Favoritism, length of experience in the relationship, native abilities, talents, and proclivities, desire and drives all play some part in determining the structure of the relationship.

As I hope you have learned by now, our master/slave relationships both have and encourage a wide variety of structures and arrangements. It is simplistic and erroneous to think that the structuring of relationships among multiple (and here I mean more than two) partners is anything but organic, meaning that the structure naturally flows from the personal characteristics, personalities, and experiences of the participants.

As a master who seeks to own multiple slaves, I prefer that they all be treated equally. Of course equal treatment does not mean they are all treated the same. I object to the notion of "alpha" because it includes the inherent idea of the superiority of one slave over others. If the "beta" slaves enjoy only passing, part-time, or limited access to the master, then there most likely will be no problems. If, on the other hand, there is the expectation of commitment, intensity, or long-term affection, then there must be equality in terms of access, pleasure, responsibility, and satisfaction. To allow otherwise is to invite doubt, feelings of inferiority, and eventual dissatisfaction. This doesn't only apply to submissives, either. Multiple masters must show respect for one another and a willingness to share freely.

This presents another caveat: when there are multiple masters there needs to be a clear delineation of authority. To note that "No man can serve two masters" is to be realistic in what is possible among humans. A slave needs the security of knowing whose orders and wishes take priority and masters must be careful not to be giving conflicting requests, as a slave can neither be in two places at the same time nor do two conflicting tasks simultaneously.

Patrick Reflects:
Who Is the Possession?

As of this writing, Sir and I have been together just over nine years. The issues most of his readers want me to respond to surround the openness of our relationship:

"Do you ever mind that Jack has other slaves and tricks?"

"Don't you get jealous when Jack has sex with others?"

"Aren't you worried that he might find someone he likes better than you?"

"How do you feel when Jack is playing with someone else?"

"Jack says he wants a lover and more slaves. Doesn't this make you angry?"

"If he loves someone else, how can he still love you?"

"When there are more slaves in the household, doesn't that mean you get less of Jack?"

I have gotten a lot of e-mail from people asking these and similar questions. Nearly every single slave-applicant worries about how I would react to him joining the household. It's the nearly universal burning subject. The topic comes up so much that Sir suggested — several times — that I should write about it for him. The truth is, it isn't all that big an issue for me. Since doing so is appropriate for this chapter, I suppose this is as good a place to start talking about it, as any.

From the start, I was seeking a master/slave relationship, not a lover relationship. Because I wanted to be owned, to have a master, I clearly accepted that much of how I lived that life would be determined by my master, not that I would determine how he lives. I certainly assumed that such a relationship would have closeness to it and an intimacy that was unique and special, but it wasn't important for me to define it as love.

I guess it helped that it wasn't my first poly relationship, but even in the previous one, I didn't think about it being non-traditional. Since everything about a Master/slave relationship is non-traditional, the number if participants involved only made it more erotic and more interesting.

Sir told me, I believe, during our first phone call that: (a) he had a lover, (b) he had a master, (c) they were not the same person, and (d) he was communicating with an additional slave-applicant. In other words, it was possible that I'd be one of two slaves. That meant that I was the second to come along. I recall that my initial reaction involved relief that it didn't put me out of the running. I probably experienced a fleeting thought that I wouldn't have him all to myself, but even then, I didn't think in terms of his being mine. I was simply content with the idea of being his.

I think this is the first erroneous idea that many people have when approaching this issue, particularly from a Master/slave perspective. Sir doesn't belong to me. A slave belongs to the Master. The idea of being owned as property by a master is one of the primary reasons someone seeks slavery; so, it should follow that prospective slaves aren't seeking to own the relationship. A slave who is certain that he must be in a monogamous relationship falls prey to the idea of "my master," as though the master belongs to the slave. Slaves belong to their masters, not the other way around. The thought of him or her as "yours" can lead the way to possessiveness, which then leads to jealousy, which breaks down trust, which affects obedience, and so on.

Slaves belong to the master. Masters don't belong to slaves. If you have trouble accepting this, do yourself a favor and admit that you really want a lover, not a master. It will save you a lot of confusion and grief in the long-run.

So, I entered the relationship with Sir knowing that, in essence, I was the outsider, the addition. The other slave never made it past the first visit. Sir's lover, Michael, lived in the western suburbs, and Master Lynn, Sir's master at the time, lived in a northern suburb; so, the fact that I was the only one living with Sir helped it work all the more smoothly.

I've often considered that a major reason why Sir and I made it through those first couple of years was that his having a lover gave me some breathing space. Sir would go out to Michael's every other weekend or so, and also after work each Tuesday, generally not returning until Wednesday night. That meant that every time some frustration built up, or the role of slave began to weigh heavily on me, I got a break for a day or two. Then, I was anxious for him to come home again.

Being in a poly relationship was seldom a chore for me.

It was also an open relationship. When we'd go out, it wasn't unusual for Sir to cruise anything within sight, often bringing someone home and sending me up to the loft while they played. Occasionally, this bothered me a bit. After a while, however, I realized that not only was I the one waking up next to his bed in the morning, I was often also the one who ended up bringing him to orgasm; he would call me down after they left or even while they were there — if things weren't going well. After all, with a trick he had to make sure they were satisfied. But with a slave, well, a slave could simply be used and then ignored.

All of the above worked well because, yes, I was flexible and not prone to jealousy, but it was also important that Sir was relatively skillful in managing the various relationships. There was an insistence on communication, and Sir followed the rules established with each partner. In general, we all supported his need to explore with each of us and with others and he worked hard to ensure that none of us felt neglected. He didn't handle all of this perfectly, but he did so with complete openness and honesty. This left no room for suspicion or doubt.

All would be for naught had I been the jealous or suspicious type. Before entering into such a rapport, I very carefully considered what I wanted in a relationship, where I felt my place would be, and what I considered acceptable and unacceptable treatment. With all of these questions answered for myself, there was little room for doubt or fear — the feelings that feed jealousy. Sir, too, was important in this. Because we were committed to the idea of a relationship of dominance and submission, he very skillfully knew how and when it should be exercised to ensure that our mutual positions remained securely in place.

Another element that allowed his exploring with others to not be a problem was that he talked about it with those whom he interviewed. When a potential addition to the family came along, we talked about both positives they might bring and potential compromises to what we had. Sir very clearly understands what we have built together, and the choice to share it with others is never done lightly. He also knows that a slave in the hand is worth two in the bush. Accordingly, he would never jeopardize our relationship for a slim possibility.

This is the second notion to consider about poly relationships. It has to be visible to all the parties involved. While the level of intimacy with a particular person might vary from time to time, each member needs to always be accessible to the others in the relationship. One reason to be in a poly relationship is that we gain different things from different people. All contribute their strengths and all can benefit from them.

I should say that most slave-applicants Sir has heard from are unsure about the idea of more than two people in a relationship, but I am never convinced that they've come to this conclusion independently. We are wired by society to think in terms of two people in a relationship as being optimal, but it's that same society that tells us that same-sex relationships are wrong or that kinky relationships are unhealthy. If you believe the latter arguments are wrong, then isn't the first one at least open to question? My suspicion is that many just assume monogamy is right for them, without clearly considering that the alternatives have a great deal to offer.

I haven't come across too many Master/slave relationships where, at some point, the master didn't develop the idea that if one slave was good, two would be even better. Relationships change over time, and it is not uncommon for a master to decide to extend the family some or at least open up the relationship. A true slave simply accepts the change, recognizing that it doesn't mean losing out; it means gaining security. If the needs in the relationship change, adjust the relationship without giving up the benefits. Stifling the changes will only lead to problems that will be more difficult to resolve later.

When I was first asked how I felt about not having my Master all to myself, I can't say I had a ready response. It's never been about having less of Sir; it's always been about retaining the quality of the relationship. For that to occur, I had to be confident that no matter who the applicants were or what role they were striving for within our family, what mattered to me was that they respected Sir and the others in our family, and respected the relationship we had developed. Respecting the relationship also means adding value to it rather than lessening its value. Over the years, there have been many who met that criteria and those that didn't, well, they didn't stay around very long.

Polyamory, open relationships, Leather family, or monogamy, go with whatever form works well for you, so long as you haven't made your choice out of ignorance. And when you are faced with the issue, don't shortchange yourself by dismissing it. In our community, these variations on the theme are just as normal for us and every bit as fulfilling as what has always been called traditional for others. And when they work and allow each member to grow and become his best, they create their own tradition.

After Reading Activities

Find three couples, one which is monogamous, one which is an open relationship, and one which is a poly arrangement of some kind.

Interview them to learn about the following:

- How do they describe their relationship?
- How did they agree upon the type of relationship they have?
- How long have they been in this relationship?
- What are the benefits and liabilities in living this way?
- How do they overcome jealousy?

Using your journal, describe each of your previous relationships and make special note of whether it was monogamous, open, or poly. What were the pros and cons of each relationship?

Ask your munch or club to sponsor a night where various kinds of relationships can be discussed, perhaps featuring speakers who are in various kinds of open or closed relationships.

Do a search on the Internet for web sites that feature poly relationships. What can you learn from these?

14

The Healthy D/s Relationship

*Erotic experiences should always contribute to the
growth of a person. S/M, if practiced correctly
and with love, does just that.*[*]

Growth is a sure sign of a healthy being and this applies to
relationships just as it does to plants, animals, and humans. Just as
relationships grow once two people meet and get to know one another,
so should they continue to grow long after their commitments are made
and their lives intertwine. Growth is, after all, a type of change and
change is the only constant that we can expect.

We often enter into relationships because of a strong attraction to
a partner whom we enjoy as they are or at least as we think they are.
Over time, though both partners will change and therefore so will their
relationship. Fostering growth in one another and in the relationship,
then, is primarily a way of insuring the future viability of the relationship.
A partnership — kinky, D/s, or otherwise — that has ceased to grow,
will soon begin to deteriorate. Time itself dictates that such is the case
and we have yet to find a way to change that.

It behooves us, then, to find ways to foster both individual and
communal growth. Committing yourselves to such a process, being open
to new ideas, pleasures, and adventures, realizing that learning about
the other is a life-long process, and being attentive to the changing
needs and desires that accompany the passage of time are all ways
to do so.

---

[*] Bannon, Race, Learning the Ropes, A Basic Guide to Safe and Fun S/M Lovemaking, Daedalus Publishing Company, Los Angeles, 1992.

The Periodic Review

Patrick and I have found that one of the best ways to encourage the health of our relationship has been to set aside a regular time devoted to doing just that. Though you and your partner may find good reason to vary the how of such a process, the fact that you value the relationship enough to reflect on it and on one another's satisfaction in it, remains extremely important.

Since the earliest days of our being master and slave, we have regularly taken time almost every Sunday evening to ask each other one simple question: "Got anything to talk about tonight?"

I routinely ask Patrick that question on at least 48 of the Sundays of a year and he asks me the same. In all honesty, the most frequent answer is "No. Do you?" I most often have nothing to say either and the discussion ends. As easy as that may seem, it affirms to each of us that our relationship is important and that we are free to speak our minds and hearts in a safe and receptive environment.

There are, to be sure, a few rules about this talk. First, we allow the other the freedom to bring up whatever he wishes and we are committed to hearing the other as best we can — without judgment, emotional reaction, or disinterest. We also recognize that doing so isn't always possible and, therefore, reserve the right to either postpone the discussion for another time (sometimes a whole week, sometimes less) or to only explore it superficially while one or both of us can work through the feeling part of the topic.

We also do our best to avoid surprises. If, for instance, there is a rather weighty topic that we are considering bringing up, we will often warn the other. Consider, for example, one Wednesday at dinner when I warned Patrick that on the forthcoming Sunday, I wished to talk about the quality of our sex life. Not coincidently, he did, too. Preparing one another for the Sunday agenda in this way, gave each of us time to consider our thoughts carefully, while preparing the other to listen to what might otherwise have been a touchy subject.

Another important parameter to the Sunday night talk is that it not be taken lightly. Therefore, we avoid having it when one of us isn't quite up to a serious discussion because of fatigue, illness, or too much partying. We never have the discussion during sex, either, as that would certainly be a difficult distraction.

We also recognize that, in this discussion, there is a need for free discourse, uninhibited by the nature of our dominant/submissive relationship. I am committed to allowing Patrick to speak freely and he understands that I respect the necessity of his doing so. In other words, there can be no threat of punishment or retaliation. We are, after all, seeking the truth, even if, for the moment, it may be difficult to hear.

We allow each other the freedom to speak on any topic and recognize that there some topics that are more difficult to broach than others; so, we allow one another the right to stumble along in getting it out and are gentle in prodding for more information or clarity. There is nothing sacred about the day, time, or frequency of our Sunday night chat, but I can assure you that the essence of regular communication fosters the kind of change that keep us individually and communally on target to achieving a healthy, lifelong relationship. This is not to say that we don't stop and talk at other times or that we only talk seriously on Sundays.

Separate Spaces

Another aspect of being together is that we recognize our need to be apart. We both have involvements outside the home that don't include the other. Patrick, for instance, is more involved with our Leather club, The Chicago Hellfire Club, while I am active in a Masonic Lodge and in the teacher's union at the college where I teach. He is an avid Star Trek fan and I an amateur genealogist. Each of us has many friends in common and a few that are certainly friends to only one of us.

We are careful, though, to keep the other informed about our lives, especially in terms of schedules, commitments, and out of the home interests. In fact, one of the rather constant questions and answers on a Sunday is a review of the commitments of the coming week, especially since knowing where we'll be and with whom determines when, how much, and what Patrick will have to cook for dinner. This reflects my belief that "No one likes surprises except on their birthday."

Separate spaces includes more than different sets of friends, different schedules, and the freedom to be apart. It also means that there is some recognition of the fact that everyone needs some time to themselves. As a night person, Patrick has the house to himself once I've fallen asleep. As an author who works alone at home, I have the place and space to myself once he's gone to work. The natural rhythms of individual lives, therefore, have made this necessity rather easy to accomplish.

One of the difficulties that the inclusion of a second slave brought upon us was that our home (a one bedroom condominium at the time) was too small for three adult men. Private spaces, then, are also a prerequisite to a healthy relationship, since they allow and encourage time to reflect, meditate, nap, and just vegetate freely — all exercises which enhance one's life. Simply put, we need to take time for ourselves so that as healthy individuals we can contribute to the health of our relationship.

Suggestions for Long-Term Relationships

Having lived in a 24/7 master/slave relationship for more than nine years, I think its durability holds some clues for doing the same with any long-term partnership. Most of the following information is just plain common sense. There is, after all, more about an M/s relationship that is human than not. What applies to everyone else applies to kinky dominants and their submissives, as well. That said, here are my suggestions.

1. Every you is plural.

This firstly refers to this section. I'm going to be using the word "you" fairly often and I'd rather not have to write "you (pl.)" every time, so remember that the yous are plural. Additionally, long-term partners have to be willing to recognize that, to some extent, they gain their partnership at the cost of their independence. A single person can think only of him or herself, a partnered one needs to think of the other you in the dynamic. In reality, members of a partnership have three entities to consider: the two individuals plus the relationship itself.

2. Know your assumptions, your expectations, and your limits.

This suggestion applies to your need to understand what you want, hope, and think, before you begin making a great deal of commitment. For better or for worse, and too often it is for the worse, we enter into a relationship because we fall in love, thereby glossing over what may be very important differences when it comes to our thoughts, our hopes, our fears, and our long range plans. We can really be suckers for the line, "Love conquers all."

The way to know these assumptions, expectations, and limits, both yours and theirs, is to discuss them freely and openly. Take some time to build a foundation for the future, lest later you end up saying, "I thought such and such" and too late learn that you thought wrongly.

3. Take time to talk.

OK, I know you're going to talk a lot with your partner. What I mean here is to set aside time to talk. Plan on having quality conversation, even when you think you don't need it. Regularly make time to check in with one another. Patrick and I do so every Sunday night. Most often the check in only takes a few seconds as we have no pressing issues. The important thing, though, is to have the time set side in case you need it. If you don't plan for it, you'll never have the time and eventually it will be too late.

4. Breathe often.

We all need space and time to ourselves so that the plural you don't strangle the individual me. Time for the individual self fosters health; so, make good use of it.

We sometimes, too, need to take a deep breath before we react to what just happened or what was just said. We often need to relax, which is easier said than done, before we make matters worse. Remember: Breathing is good; do it often. It's like counting to ten before you blow up.

5. Create special moments.

Take time to cherish one another, even if the time is a short one. Flowers, candy, cards, and almost any bit of thoughtfulness go a long way, a very long way, in preserving and improving your long-term relationship. Too often, we take each other for granted. A pat on the ass, a kiss on the cheek, or a thank you does just the opposite. Try it. You'll both like it.

6. Be yourself and let your partner do the same.

A long-term relationship doesn't mean that you have plenty of time to change the other person into what you want him to be. Start your relationship on the basis of your honest self expressing its true nature. If you can't do that, then go find a partnership where you can.

7. Encourage, empower and give to facilitate change.

LTRs, since they are long-term, mean that change is inevitable. Stand by your (wo)man. Allow him or her to grow, learn, and develop. Expect change and do your best to make the changes for the better.

8. Put your commitment in writing.
Review and revise it periodically.

Ever since the Tower of Babel, it's been difficult for us to really understand one another. Putting thoughts on paper does make them clearer. Added to the gained clarity is the fact that a mark of ink on a piece of paper remembers a lot more precisely than any amount of brain cells. The troth you pledge today will not be repeated the same way a year from now unless you write it down.

That said, you may find it necessary to change what you wrote. That's life. Neither of you will be the same person in the relationship as time goes on; so, it's only realistic to review what you have written and mutually agree to change it to fit the new (and we hope better) you.

9. Don't hide your relationship, but don't scare
the natives with it either.

Since we're talking about kinky relationships, we may have the idea that we need to keep them secret. We don't and we probably shouldn't. On the other hand you can always call a significant other a partner, a

259

friend, or a pal. The world doesn't need to know what you do in your bedroom. There is an appropriate time and place for everything, but every time and place may not be appropriate.

10. Remember to have fun.

As partners, you will cry, work, worry, and plan together. The drudgery of everyday living will always be there; therefore, make time to have fun and keep it as one of your objectives. If you're not laughing with each other once in a while, something is amiss. Find out why and plan for smiles. Fun is important! Make it so.

The Unspoken Reality

As I finished writing this book, I began thinking of an appropriate and inspirational ending and I decided to write about love between master and slave. So I did a word count and found that I used the word "love" or one of its variant forms less than 50 times in a manuscript of more than 95,000 words. "What does that say about love in mastery and slavery?" I asked myself.

Reflecting on my own query, I remembered the many discussions I've had over the years, repeated in chat rooms and newsgroups, I'm sure, about whether masters and slaves can, should, or do love one another. The usual answer varies across the spectrum: yes, no, sometimes, in some ways, maybe, yes for the slave and no for the master, etc., etc., etc.

The question is compounded by the wide variation in the way we use the word "love." It's a sad fact that the English language is much too vague in its usage and meaning of the word "love." After all, there are many kinds of love and the manifestations of each of them is certainly quite different from one definition to another. We love parents, children, sex partners, chocolate, life, movies, songs, friends, uncles, cousins, and our careers — each in its own way.

What compounds the discussion of love between kinky associates — be they masters and slaves, tops and bottoms, husbands and wives, significant others, good friends and fuck-buddies, etc. — is that each of these pairings can be held together by many qualities; love is only one of them. When love, however you mean the term, is a quality in a kinky relationship, it too may widely vary in nature from one set of partners to another. There's nothing to say, for instance, that one sadomasochistic couple has to share the same kind of love as another.

Still I wondered about the lack of love in my manuscript. In continued reflection, it was obvious that the master/slave couples who I know best did, in fact, love one another, though to call them lovers lent a decidedly inaccurate view to their relationship. In a similar way, calling a married couple lovers seems to be somewhat presumptive, even though one would hope that they were, in fact, in love with each other and loved one another and based their relationship on love.

I asked a slave-applicant, who has been coming around for about six weeks, if he loved me. He hesitated in his answer. I understand that hesitation very well, as life experience has a way of changing one's appreciation of the value of "falling in love." Is that because we view love differently as we mature? Is there something about romance that loses its charm as we age? Is emotional love — as in Romeo and Juliet — something only for the young or the foolish? Does love lose its ardor because we become wise or because we become jaded?

In my continued reflection, I realized that a similar count of the frequency of the word "air" in my manuscript would show that I only used it once, unless you also count the number of times it appears joined with the word plane, as in "airplane." I then breathed a sigh of relief.

Love permeates our relationships in the same way that air permeates our lives. It is ubiquitous and essential to them. Love is everywhere, but seldom noticed. Just as we speak of air in terms of its manifestations, so, too, we talk not of love, as much as we speak of its effects.

Just as the air is windy or cold or breezy or smelly or pleasant, love is affectionate, caring, careful, attentive, devoted, enthralling, captivating, wonderful, trusting, concerned, pleasurable, or intimate. We see not love itself but its effect. We talk not about loving one another but of how we love. Very often, too, we don't even speak about how we love. Instead we just do it, as simply as we breathe.

Patrick's first letter to me, for instance, contained the telling phrase, "I do not seek a lover." We began our relationship without love, and for the first several years when I asked Patrick if he loved me, he would only reply that he loved being my slave.

The basis of our relationship was domination and obedience; responses to our individual awareness concerned who we were, what we needed, and what we wanted. We liked one another, to be sure. We clicked right away as master and slave. Together, we found great pleasure in the other, but we were not lovers. It may even be safe to say that we have never fallen in love with each other either, as that romantic, emotional response has never seemed to be part of our lives.

Do we love one another? That is another question. Shall I count the ways? Like the air we breathe, it permeates our lives together. Friends see it readily in how we treat each other. We know it well, as we manifest it in concern, in affection, in devotion, in the ever-tightening bonds that unite us as partners, as a couple, as friends, as fuck-buddies, and kinky players, as joint home owners, and as life-mates.

We are well past the ninth anniversary of the day we met, and the night when we knew we were somehow "made" for each other.

That understanding of belonging has never left. It has changed only in quality, as day after day, the bonds tightened, the intimacy grew, and affection prospered, our love deepened.

I once conducted a weekend workshop on mastery and slavery at the end of which I was challenged to "go home and tell Patrick you love him." I accepted that challenge, as it was an easy one — though simply saying "I love you" doesn't give much indication of what I meant. He is best friend, spouse, partner, delightful slave, devoted assistant, faithful servant, protective and watchful guard, excellent cook and careful provider. He supports, advises, performs innumerable household chores, encourages, critiques, caresses, satisfies, nurtures, and even worships.

Is there love? How can it not be seen? How can it not be there? Still, like the air, it is best noted in its effect: a sweet, vital, essential, refreshing, sustaining, and necessary element so clear as to be invisible and so fundamental as to be overlooked.

It's easy to miss that fact that love is present, just as we take the air we breathe for granted. Still it is a many splendored essential. Take a deep breath and be thankful for it. Tell those you love that such is so.

In Summary

The simplest way to take the mystery out of master/slave relationships is to recognize that they are human relationships. In many aspects, they differ little from relationships at work, in marriage, between friends and lovers. Let your life be ordered by common sense, empowered by self-knowledge, and spiced with fantasy. Together, those characteristics will put you in good stead as you and your partner create your otherwise unique relationship.

Patrick Reflects: Relationship Survival

Master/slave relationships are often thought of as being odd, or strange, out of the norm, or not true relationships. Let's put it into perspective. Dictionaries can vary in the amount of words spent on "relationship," but common to all that I consulted was the idea of involvement. It could be as specific as blood-related or marriage, or as loose as having things in common, or as distinctive as emotional relationships or sexual relationships.

With that in mind, then, we can say that bitter enemies have relationships. Married couples going through divorce disputes have relationships — often with a relationship continuing afterwards — much to their dismay. Dysfunctional families have relationships. Prisoners and jailers have relationships. Doctors and patients have relationships. Parents and children have relationships. Relationships are a common occurrence of life, and given the wide range of strange bedfellows who have them, it's a wonder that Master/slave relationships are considered strange, rather than normal.

When people think "relationship," they assume something fulfilling, happy-making and ongoing; so, there is a critical distinction between having a relationship and having a healthy relationship. The fact is that most people don't recognize being locked into an unhealthy relationship until it is crumbling in their grasp. It doesn't have to be that way. All it takes is to stop and look at it with an open mind from time to time.

Here are some very basic relationship ideas that you've heard before. Heck, everyone has heard them before, but they often dismiss them as "yes, I know that" pieces of information. But each time you have to listen to them, you have another opportunity to take them more to heart and apply them. So, don't skip over them thinking you already know them; they always bear repeating, and in this case, with a little slant to allow for our lifestyle.

A healthy D/s relationship is allowed to foster growth and change.

We all mature over time; it's a part of life. When we are content and fulfilled, change faces less resistance and generally happens without our realizing it. The things that began your master/slave relationship have to adjust with them. Events will change how you look at yourself, your master, and at things, in general. If slavery causes you to thrive as a person (which it should), change is inevitable. Being owned by another doesn't make you immune to that.

These changes might involve sex, play, rituals or even time together. Some of the dynamics your master/slave relationship revolve around are foundational and will always create that same thrill as the very first time, while others will grow commonplace, and even boring, over time. There always has to be room for new experiences and this is the responsibility of both the master and the slave. Sometimes, merely the affirmation or reinforcement of what's important and basic is all that's necessary. The key is in knowing what is still important to the other and to allow for that, and what's worth bringing in that's new and exciting to both.

Your relationship must adjust to changes gradually and proactively. Otherwise, you'll wake up one morning and realize you just aren't happy with the way things are. You'll begin spending a great deal of energy trying to recapture what you had. Once it's gone, however, you can't bring back the past, no matter how hard you try.

The relationship IS going to change, but it doesn't have to leave out the master/slave dynamic. Move with change and find ways for it to define and enhance what you already have, and it will keep your relationship healthy and ready to embrace more change.

A healthy D/s relationship is one where communication freely moves back and forth between Master and slave.

The Master dominates and the slave obeys. That's the nature of the relationship. Many strive for extremes in this dynamic. This acquiescence can carry over into most parts of the relationship, making for some very erotic living.

Dominance should not overtake communication. Communication IS a power exchange, and shouldn't be relegated to an unimportant segment of the relationship. A slave is a thinking, feeling, human being, and if communication doesn't flow back and forth, the slave isn't going to be functioning at his best. When a slave harbors unspoken issues and feelings, hurt feelings, misunderstandings, or questions, any and all of these things interfere with the slave's ability to serve, obey and submit.

Communication happens on a variety of levels: body language, actions, words, feelings, heart, mind, but they have to have an outlet and it doesn't become "communication" until it is acknowledged. I can listen for hours on end, but unless I hear what you are saying, then we haven't communicated.

A slave isn't a simple automaton. Though some seem to strive for this fantasy, it's sure to be an unhealthy one if lived out in real-time. While your master might not communicate with his toaster, he probably doesn't stick his dick into it, either. Unquestioned obedience and submission might be the ongoing occurrence in your relationship, but make sure there is time for communication.

A healthy D/s relationship thrives on honesty and openness.

Sometimes you don't realize a relationship is going to develop from an interaction with someone, leading you to fudge facts. It seems innocent and harmless ("everybody does it") and it makes breaking the ice easier for you. As a relationship evolves, though, at some point the inconsistencies come back to haunt you and you are faced with the harder decision of how to handle them. It's sometimes a matter of being tripped up by them or trapped because your partner becomes aware of them. Either way, it's obvious that there was a breach of trust.

Depending upon the untruths, or the amount of them, such issues can often be overcome; since they remain a faint ghost in the relationship, it's far better to not have the problem to be begin with. If it's your habit to embellish truths or play games with your profile, break the habit. It won't serve you well in a relationship, particularly in a master/slave relationship, where a much greater degree of control is given to the master.

Trust is what defines a relationship. Think of an open meadow with rolling hills. You can run through them, oblivious of everything, but one day you come across someone special and you want to stop and get to know the person better. You pick up a stone and set it down as a marker — something to keep track of your beginnings. That stone is your first bit of trust — that the person also might want to get to know you better.

Over time, the stones pile up, building a little wall that defines a space, a relationship, a special place a little removed from the rest of the meadow. As the relationship grows, the wall is strengthened and even enlarged. When adversity hits, it weathers it. Even if a few stones get knocked away, there are many more that help hold it together. If the relationship is long and healthy, there are lots of stones, each individually placed and each one a token of some trust developed, each one having a special meaning.

Of course, if the stones get knocked away faster than they can be replaced, that special place ceases to exist.

A healthy D/s relationship provides space for each person to be himself.

In the beginning, you won't be able to get enough of your master. The sex will be hot. You will think of each other constantly. You want to be everything he wants you to be. A lot of effort gets expended planning time together, as you each explore the other, as you each learn what the other can give and take. There's a special energy that happens when a relationship is being tried. It's the kind that can build closeness for the long-term.

This magical period reveals the special nature each of you has, and that uniqueness is largely what enthralled you each with the other in the first place. Pledges of obedience and submission notwithstanding, you have to hold onto the essence of that special person who existed before you gave yourself to another.

One way of doing this is to be sure you are you. It's much easier and much more fun to be you than to pretend to be something or someone else. Sooner or later, it catches up anyway. Trust me! Healthy relationships are made of real people, not manufactured images!

Another is to follow Shakespeare's advice from *Hamlet*: "This above all; to thine own self be true." (Act I, scene iii). Slaves, particularly, are prone to submerge themselves and their needs into the desires and wants of their masters. Don't forget to please yourself.

You also need to continue to grow as a person. "When we learn nothing new about ourselves in a relationship that's when the relationship is over. Or it's over the moment when we're afraid to learn something new about ourselves."[†] You don't lose yourself in slavery; you recreate

† Robinson, Andrew J., *A Stitch in Time*

yourself, keeping all of the most interesting parts.

A healthy D/s relationship is a process.

Sometimes, it looks like everyone else does it better. You go to an event and you notice those who do things differently, or seemingly better. Perhaps you envy how they seem to be a touch more obedient, a bit quicker to respond, more attentive. Maybe you envy how they are decked out or how hard their owners use them in the dungeon. What you need to remember is that this lifestyle is a process. There is no instant slavery. You learn as you go, and you learn as your master trains you. Not every master wants the same attributes in a slave and not every slave could serve your master the way you can. You'll learn what you need as you go along. Your only concern should be to learn your lessons well.

You'll also realize that many of those same people will be observing you, as well, and envious of you in their own ways.

Healthy D/s relationships naturally keep getting better.

After Reading Activities

How well do you communicate? Does your style need improvement? Can you find some resources that might help? Look for them, list them in your journal, and take advantage of at least one of them.

How did your past relationships end? What do you think went wrong and why? What do you think you have to change in your life to prevent the same thing from happening again?

Do you have the following tools to help you in your search?

- Description of what you want to be and how you imagine your slavery.
- What will your future life look like?
- An ad seeking a master.
- A list of places where you can place your ad and where you can find masters' personal ads, as well.
- The questionnaire in Appendix B, with your answers. (Questions may be modified to suit your specific needs/vision.)
- A blank questionnaire for your master-applicant.
- A petition to serve.
- A sample of the contract you will sign.
- A list of things to do to get ready for slavery.
- A realistic timetable for enthrallment.

How complete is your slave portfolio? Isn't it about time you started getting it ready or started to use it? Good luck!

A Necessary Last Word

I've finished writing and you've finished reading, unless you're the kind of reader who first goes to the back of the book to learn its ending. It is my sincere hope that I've explained an exciting and rewarding relationship to you.

I also trust that you now have the information and the tools you need to find the master or mistress with whom you will create a special — and yes, loving — relationship.

If that's not the case, I encourage you to start over, to practice what I am preaching: know yourself and commit yourself to the search. Persevere in the search until you have that which you seek.

I wish you luck, courage, and most of all, love.

Jack Rinella
Chicago
December 2004

Appendix A:
Glossary

Please note that this glossary is not intended to be a complete dictionary of terms used by kinky folks, only a guide to understanding the vocabulary of a master/slave relationship. All definitions are my definitions and each word may, in fact, be defined or used by others in a different way. I have purposefully not included those terms which are used with the meaning found in a standard dictionary, as to do so would most likely violate copyright laws.

24/7/365   24 days a week, seven days a week, every day of the year.

Applicant   One applying for a position not yet achieved, either as master or slave.

Apprentice   One learning from another in order to be in a relationship with someone else.

Body worship   The worship, praise, and adoration of a master or of the master's body by his or her slave. This is often a euphemism for oral (as compared to vocal) sexual pleasuring of the dominant

Boi   The feminine and/or African-American version of boy.

Bondage   A popular fetish that uses various forms of restraint, especially rope, leather and chains.

Bottom   The one on the passive or receiving end of an activity; one who prefers to receive.

Boy   A person who defines him or herself as such. It is a very self-defined role and may be dominant or submissive.

Coming out   A life-long process that involves acknowledging one's sexual orientation, though it can also be applied to admitting one's kinky sexual activities as well.

Contract   An essay defining the agreement determining a master/slave relationship usually signed by both parties.

Control	The ability to direct.
D/s	An abbreviation for Dominant/submissive.
Daddy	A person in a relationship that is marked by mentoring and protection of another person.
Discipline	When used in its kinky form, the use of impact tools (whips, crops, paddles, etc) in order to inflict pain for the purpose of giving pleasure to the recipient.
Domestic Violence	Abusive and non-consensual activity imposed by one partner on the other.
Dominant	A personality trait for a person who naturally takes control, leads, or directs. Note that I try not use this word as referring to a person but rather to a particular characteristic. Dom is the male form, Domme, the female, though they are pronounced the same (since they are taken from the French).
Domination	Exercising a high degree of control of another.
Edge Play	Any fetish that borders on danger, such as those involving blood or breath control.
Enthrallment	The process of becoming a slave; enslavement.
Family	A self-identified group, more or less structured that provides mutual support and encouragement.
Guardian Master	A person who mentors, supervises, or advises a slave wannabe either until the wannabe finds a master or in the absence of a master.
Guardian Slave	A person who is under the direction of a Guardian Master.
Kinky	Any sexual relationship that includes BDSM — that is, bondage, discipline (whipping, spanking, and other impact fetishes), dominance, submission, sadism, and masochism.
Leather Bar	A retail establishment that serves alcohol and primarily caters to a kinky clientele, especially but not exclusively or always, composed of Gay Leathermen.
Leather	Generally, a euphemism for any and all kinds of kinky relationships, including BDSM, D/s, and alternate lifestyles. Specifically it applies to the culture of Gay kinky men.
Leatherman	A gay man who is kinky.
Limit	An activity that is out of bounds, i.e., one in which one of the participants will not participate, such as whipping to blood or unsafe sex.
Long-term	Lasting more than a year.
M/s	An abbreviation for master/slave.

Masochism	The enjoyment of receiving consensual pain.
Masochist	One who finds sexual pleasure in receiving certain kinds of pain.
Master	One who controls and is obeyed by one who has surrendered his or her life to the master. Please note that I use the word "master" to apply to a specific gender.
Mistress	The feminine form of master.
Monogamy	A sexual relationship limited to one couple.
Munch	A public meeting of kinky folks, usually held at a restaurant as a safe way for online people to meet. The munches are a place to find play partners, learn about groups, and become part of a real-time and place community.
Pansexual	Open to all sexes, genders and orientations.
Petition	The request, usually written, to enter into a master/slave relationship for service or training.
Play Party	A gathering of kinky folk, usually sponsored by a club, organization, or munch in order to provide a safe space for kinky activity.
Polyamory	A sexual relationship that includes more than two partners.
Professional Dominatrix	A woman who provides D/s experiences for a fee. In rarer cases such is provided by a male called a Professional Dominator.
Protocols	The individualized forms of ceremony and etiquette that a slave is required by his or her master to perform.
Punishment	Any negative reinforcement imposed by a master in response to the slave's disobedience.
Reference	A person who will vouch for another. One who will verify a person's experience, information, or trustworthiness to some degree.
Rimming	Oral/anal contact, especially licking the anus with the tongue.
Sadism	The enjoyment of the consensual infliction of pain.
Sadist	One who derives sexual pleasure from the infliction of pain, though not of injury.
Sadomasochistic	Having both sadistic and masochistic characteristics.
Safe Word	An agreed upon word that will stop an activity. At times there are three safe words in a relationship, one for slow down and one for stop and resume, and one for stop altogether.
Service	An act of obedience.

Slave-in-Training A person who is not yet in a long-term, committed relationship of slavery, but who is learning to be so enslaved.

Slave The state in which a person chooses to be in a relationship of obedience and service to another. This is actually shorthand for one who is in the condition of Voluntary Servitude.

Stable A reference to a group of slaves under the control of a master.

Submissive The personality trait in which a person prefers to receive, obey, or serve.

Surrender The release of oneself, especially one's body and will, to the control of another.

Top The role assumed by the active player. Also refers to one who prefers that role.

Trainee One learning from a mentor, from a person who is simply a casual teacher, or from one who is preparing the other to enter into a relationship with him or her.

Voluntary Servitude A more appropriate name for the relationship in our subculture commonly called a slavery.

Wannabe A person with no connection to a master but who is considering slavery as a life option.

Worship The vocal praise and adoration of a master by his or her slave, akin to that which is given to a god.

Appendix B:

Guidelines for a Questionnaire

The following ideas are presented so that you will have an outline to facilitate the creation of your own questionnaire.

Personal Data:
Full Name, Address, City, State, Zip, Phone number
Age, Height, Weight, Waist size, Color and amount of hair
Education level
Occupation, Title, How long at your present job?

Are you single, partnered, married, divorced. For how long? Describe your previous relationships.
Is your relationship open, monogamous, polyamorous?

Health
List any health conditions that you have.
What medications do you take?
What are your personal guidelines concerning safer sex?

Family
Are your parents living?
How many brothers and sisters do you have?
Are you in contact with them?
To what extent do they know of your participation in an alternate lifestyle?

Finances
In general terms what do you earn in a year?
How large is your debt?
Do you have savings?
Can you afford to travel?

Fetishes
Shaving, feet, ass play, bondage, whipping, cross-dressing, water sports, scat, piercing (temporary and permanent), spanking, slapping, clothespins and clamps, verbal abuse, enemas, fisting, pony/puppy play, leather, rubber, vinyl, wrestling

Sex
Fucking, sucking, rimming, cuddling, kissing, solos and three-ways

Drug use
Alcohol, Dope, Poppers, Meth, Speed, Coke, Cigarettes, Coffee

Relationship issues
What do you seek in a master?
What do you offer as a slave?
What are your D/s experiences?
Why do you think you are a slave?
What are your thoughts on control, obedience, worship, service?

What kind of a relationship are you seeking in terms of:
Length, intensity, domestic activities, part-time/full-time/occasional

Describe your readiness or when you think you will be ready.
Are you willing to consider relocating?

Appendix C

Expectations and Regulations concerning

Voluntary Servitude

(Please note that you're welcome to copy this and use it, but please let your friends know you got it from *Becoming a Slave* by Jack Rinella.) This document sets out the ramifications of surrendering one's life to mastery.

PREREQUISITES

The onset of slavery begins once several conditions have been met. As shown here, they are *sine qua non* — that is, without them, Voluntary Servitude cannot proceed.

1.   The slave will demonstrate full knowledge of the ramifications of surrender and will accept the conditions of such without reservation or hesitation. It must be perfectly clear to both parties that it is a free, informed, and adult choice to enter into the relationship of voluntary servitude (henceforth referred to as "slavery"). Submission to this lifestyle under the dominance and control of a master must be a free choice entered into by the slave without coercion or deceit.

2.   The master will do his best to clarify the meaning, implications, and impact of slavery. On the slave's part, he must be willing to allow full knowledge of his person to his master. This demands an openness and intimacy on the slave's part so that control over him can be complete, informed, and in the best interests of the master.

3.   There needs to be a trial period of slavery to insure full understanding of the master's conditions, requirements, and expectations. The master will use this trial time to evaluate at close range the slave's appropriateness, motivations, and attitude.

4.   Throughout the slave's subjugation, he will demonstrate the following characteristics:

an eagerness to learn what is expected of him as slave and to fulfill those expectations;

an attitude that demonstrates the need and desire to be dominated;

a response to the master's commands, suggestions, and desires that proves his desire to please, serve, and live in a way that will meet the master's conditions.

5.   The master will provide for the slave's needs out of the slave's present and future resources and income. This provision will be according to the master's allocation, not the slave's.

GENERAL PRINCIPLES

The rules of service may be summarized by four core statements defining the slave's position:
1.   Respect at all times.
2.   Surrender of physical control over all parts of the slave's body.
3.   The acceptance of discipline without complaint or resistance.
4.   The attitude of thankfulness for whatever attention is bestowed by the master.

The following pages expand these rules and apply them to the definition of a complete lifestyle.

THE MASTER'S RESPONSIBILITIES

1.   He will respect the slave's need to fulfill certain obligations inherent in life, e.g., issues of health, nutrition, family obligations, occupation, finances, etc. Once slavery is begun, decisions in matters such as these will be made by the master, not by the slave. For obvious reasons they may have the appearance of being the slave's decisions.

Since the slave has chosen to be controlled, the master's decisions will be the slave's decisions in a very real (albeit indirect) way. As necessary, the master may include the slave in the decision-making process, but only with the recognition that the slave's role will be one of advice, not direction, nor will it involve the slave in reclaiming decision-making authority for himself, except when specifically granted by the master.

2.   Once the slave is the master's property, the master will be responsible to keep him as healthy as possible. The master will want to keep his property at full value and so will not command or treat the

slave in a way that jeopardizes or diminishes his value. A healthy slave is a valuable one.

THE RAMIFICATIONS OF SLAVERY

Appearance
The slave will look as most pleases the master in matters of grooming, dress, decorum, manners, and outward demeanor.

Behavior Modification
The master will use, and the slave will assent to the use of, behavior modification techniques. Once the slave is under the master's control, certain changes in the slave's behavior may be required so that the slave conforms more exactly to the master's will.

Techniques will include (but are not limited to) discipline, deprivation, instruction, positive reinforcement, encouragement, incentives, isolation, and reward.

Conflict
The slave will submit to the master's judgment in the (likely) event that there arises conflict between them. In the case of conflict, the slave can expect the application of behavior modification, discipline, dialogue, and honesty.

Continued Ownership
The termination of the master's ownership of the slave will be at the master's pleasure, and in light of the slave's constitutional rights (see below). The master's continued ownership of the slave will be at the master's pleasure and the master reserves the right to transfer the slave's ownership to another person either temporarily or permanently at the master's discretion.

Dialogue
The master will provide the slave with opportunities to express the slave's needs and discuss the slave's concerns. The master will listen to the slave, endeavoring to teach him, and as appropriate, help the slave understand the master's actions. There will be the opportunity for questioning and discussion, always though in the context that the master is the decision maker and the master alone holds final say.

The master's willingness to inform the slave and help the slave understand is at the master's discretion. The slave has no need to understand, unless the master perceives that such understanding will improve the slave's worth and service to him.

Discipline

As stated above the slave will receive discipline for the master's pleasure and the slave's training. The master will teach the slave to accept it willingly and totally. The slave will be open to it and will find the inner strength and commitment to transform the negative aspects of discipline (pain, humiliation, discomfort, trauma, etc.) into a positive viewpoint and eventually as a natural, expected, and welcome aspect of the slave's submission.

Discipline will not be administered in such a way as to injure the slave nor decrease the slave's value. It will be an integral part of the slave's lifestyle, according to the master's direction and will.

The master will use hands, paddles, belts, cat-o-nine tails, brushes, confinement, bondage, deprivation, or other means suitable to help the slave acquire and maintain appropriate attitudes and responses.

Duties

The slave will work as directed by the master in order to provide income for both himself and his master.

The slave will perform duties appropriate to the slave's schedule, health and capacity, such as housekeeping, volunteer work, errands, etc., in the service of his master.

There will be a published schedule of chores, responsibilities, and expectations, as determined by the master and subject to his supervision, control, and modification.

Emancipation

In respect for the Constitution and laws of the United States of America, the master recognizes that coercion is neither a viable nor legal means of enforcing the slave's submission. Hence the slave will be in a condition of Voluntary Servitude, that is, the slave's slavery depends upon the slave's recognition of his need to be dominated and owned. In fact, the slave's own will creates and maintains this slavery.

Fear and related obstructions

An important part of the slave's growth and development will be the elimination, by trial, experience, experiment, submission, and obedience, of blocks and hindrances to the slave's full service to the master's will. Characteristics such as fear, doubt, insecurity, and hesitancy will be eliminated by encouragement, training, discipline and direct confrontation.

In this process the slave will be stripped of all limits, excuses, inner restraint, superficiality, false modesty, and phobias. Instead the slave will submit to the limits the master imposes upon the slave, with confidence in the master's ability to control the slave's life and actions.

It is expected that the degree of submission will be such that the slave will rely on the master without hesitation or reservation, knowing that all justifiable and necessary limits will be kept by the master in light of the master's protection of his property.

Finances

Upon entry into servitude, the slave will turn practical and actual (but not legal) control of his personal resources over to the master for administration.

Assets will remain the property of the slave. Nothing in this section is meant to imply that the master is using the relationship for his own self-aggrandizement. Similarly this is not a "free ride" for the slave.

The master will administer the slave's finances in such a way as to increase their value and provide for the slave's present and future needs (see section on The master's RESPONSIBILITIES).

The slave will support himself and provide for the master's pleasure and prosperity. The master will not accept the role of providing for the slave — as that would in fact make him the slave's slave, a role the master is not willing to accept. As the master's property the slave will not be allowed to become a drain on the master's finances, but rather an asset to them.

Honesty

The slave will be open, frank and honest in his conversation and relationship with the master. Any breach of this confidence will invoke the use of discipline.

Housing

The slave will live in the domicile of his master's choosing, either in the master's home or in close proximity to it, as the master sees fit. It will be open to the master's inspection and use at all times. The slave will respect the master's space as private and the slave's presence in it as one of slave and servant, performing such duties as ordered at the time and in the manner so commanded.

The type and location of the slave's place of residence shall be according to the master's assignment and within the range of the master's allocation of the slave's resources.

Sexual Behavior

It is understood that sexual intimacy will be part of the master/slave relationship. It will be conducted at all times as directed by the master's will and pleasure. The slave's sexual activity will be under the master's control. It is recognized that the objective of the slave's submission is the master's pleasure, not the slave's, though the slave may find his duties in this area pleasurable.

At all times the slave will adhere to the practice of safe sex, as defined by the master.

Social Life

At the master's discretion, the slave will be given the opportunity to experience a social life outside of the master's supervision, though any absences from the master's service will be with the master's prior approval.

The master will expect and encourage the slave to develop other friendships, interests, and relationships. The only qualification of this is that they will not compete for the master's attention or time.

As the master desires and instructs, the slave will be made to treat others as the slave's master *pro tem*. Likewise, the slave will be expected to assist the master in the instruction, domination, and pleasurable use of other slaves. The master does not expect the slave to take a role of domination, but rather one of facilitation.

IN SUMMARY

This, then, describes the slave's servitude, though it by no means fully describes the actual ramifications of the slave's submission. How it is lived out actually will be shown by time, the master's decisions, and the slave's submission.

A list of rules is appended for your information and memorization.

1. I will address my master with respect at all times, referring to him as either "master" or "Sir".
2. I will keep my legs spread apart for his pleasure at all times.
3. As his slave I recognize his control over all parts of my body and therefore I will not touch my body — which is his — without permission nor will I perform any bodily movement or function without his command to do so.
4. I will accept discipline willingly, knowing that my master is in control and has more wisdom, knowledge, and experience than I in these matters.
5. I will remain thankful for my master's attention — whether it be painful or pleasurable — and will thank him for such attention as appropriate.

Appendix D:

An Interview with Patrick

Sir suggested that I consider making a contribution to this book and in the beginning I was a bit reluctant. It wasn't that I didn't think I had something to contribute because this kind of relationship has brought out the best in me, given me more, and has caused me to grow more, I think, than all of the previous 40 years that came before. But it takes me a while to crank out coherent thoughts that hang together well. My friend David Stein does it effortlessly, grammar-perfect and logically but I have to work at being that carefully thought-provoking. I wasn't sure how my thoughts would flow and worried that they'd come back to haunt me, but ultimately I decided that I did have something to say and began to frame it out.

In the meantime Sir decided try to encourage me on the idea and came up with this list of questions I could answer that could be my contribution. "You don't need to say a lot," he said, "just answer the questions. A couple of paragraphs each". The problem was that I didn't know how to break it to him that I had already decided to say a lot. I didn't want him to think I was taking over his book. (Masters, after all, are supposed to be the ones in control.)

In the end I took the list of questions but worked on my contributions in my own way. Answering the list of questions was quite valid and a lot could be said through them. Interviews were the beginning point for this book and I realized Sir never did a formal one with me. So I began answering them to see what would come of them.

Sir: How did you first discover the idea of masters and slaves?
It was 1978. I was a junior and a ministerial student in a small private Christian college in southeast Kentucky and was driving our church pianist home to St. Louis for Christmas break. I had just dropped her off and got back on the highway when the bottom fell out of the

clouds and it rained so hard that I couldn't see the road ahead. It was late afternoon and I didn't think I could make the 5 or 6 hour trip back to school, given the storm, so I turned back towards St. Louis, creeping along, crossed the river, and found an exit that had a motel to stay in for the night.

I checked in and, of course, the storm stopped, and it wasn't long before I was bored in a strange, unfamiliar town. It was too late at that point to get back on the road so I got in the car to find a movie theater or something to do. The motel was not far from the river and my driving took me into what is now the touristy Busch Stadium area. It wasn't back then. There wasn't a movie theater anywhere to be found and there wasn't a shopping area where I could find a good book to read, nothing, except for an adult book store. I'd never been in an adult bookstore before, and I was bored enough to be curious.

It really wasn't that simple. I was sexually confused, didn't really know why I wasn't interested in girls as more than friends and I was afraid to think about what that meant. I was worried that people would somehow find out about my secret, my fantasies, what I jerked off thinking about so it was best not to think about it at all. But it wasn't easy not to think about it... at least the fantasies.

So I went into the adult bookstore to satisfy my curiosity, thinking, perhaps, I might also find something that would satisfy my confusion. I did, but not in the way I expected.

The walls were covered in magazine racks holding heterosexual porn. I'd never dreamed there was such a variety of smut; it was everywhere. But it wasn't the walls I was drawn to; and the truth is, I didn't want to be. Just across from the door, as though they knew I needed it to be easily found, was a rack that had a sign above it that read "GAY". Who would have thought that an adult bookstore would have a gay section? I hadn't even considered there was anything to have a Gay section for. But without even thinking about it that's where I headed and I picked up the first thing within my reach that looked safe: *Drummer Magazine, issue 32.*

Except it didn't have anything to do with drummers.

I was in a daze as I flipped through its pages, not even paying attention to what was on them until my eyes fell on a full page image of what would change my entire life: the illustration of a collared Jamie, kneeling and looking up at an unseen Mr. Benson with that worshipful, submissive gaze.

It was as though everything made sense at that moment, all of the questions in my mind about who I was, what I wanted in life, and why normal didn't feel normal for me. I didn't think twice. I had to have that magazine. I started to go and pay for it right then but as I turned to find out where to pay I saw "Action Male", and "Bound to Serve" and "S&M with Steve and Marty." I left with several treasures, and hurried back to the motel where I read and jerked off more times than I could keep track of.

Sir: What do you and Jack have in common?
It's an interesting mix, I suppose. There is a lot more we complement each other on than we have in common. He's a morning person and I'm night person, which gives us each some quiet time alone. He thrives with roller coaster emotions, while I am fairly even-keeled; so, we can move through issues without going over the edge. He gets caught up in the spur of the moment and I find ways of fitting it into the plan or adjusting the plan accordingly.

I wasn't as strong-willed at the beginning of the relationship as I guess I am now; so, I did the proper slave thing and tried to let my Master determine as much of my life as possible and that's worked pretty well for us. Even so, we wouldn't have lasted if there hadn't been some commonalities to steady the fledgling relationship.

We are both content to spend quiet evenings at home a lot. We also share similar preferences when it comes to eating. Neither of us is materialistic or big on shopping. We don't watch much TV but we read a lot so we are comfortable keeping ourselves entertained... no pun intended. We agree on most community and political issues, approach things in differently but usually on roughly parallel paths, and we both like sex to be edgy. There are a lot of little things that can punch little holes in a relationship but we had a good foundation to build the kinky stuff on.

Sir: How did you discover your call to serve?
For me it isn't a call to serve, perhaps because I was convinced that I'd been called to serve in the ministry, and that I view the idea of a "call" as something you just convince yourself of, without really knowing what to do with it. It's much too simple to give in without testing it, and you end up letting others put you on a predetermined path.

My slavery does contain some altruism, but it has to contain much more than that to keep me choosing to serve. No, it wasn't a call, it's much better than that.

Sir: How did you decide to become Jack's slave?
Luck of the draw, I think.
Actually it was very easy, far easier than most have it. Though we were both strangers he'd had a lot of his thoughts published, and these allowed me, over time as I read them, to gain a sense of who he was.

His writing contains a great deal of self-refection and reveals a great deal about him, even when it isn't obvious, so each time I'd encountered something he'd written I was getting to know him a bit better.

I also considered that, since he was a public figure, he'd have to be genuine. If he talked the talk, so to speak, but didn't walk the walk, his reputation would have suffered, he'd have lost his audience and lost the opportunity to write for the public. By the time I'd met him I knew him pretty well.

I don't know whether I felt that he was the right one as I crossed the door of his home that first afternoon but later that night there was little question. We'd clicked on many levels as the evening wore on and by the time we were playing it was a foregone conclusion.

That's not to say there weren't second thoughts at times. As soon as the next few days I had doubts. Once he began seeing how intensely I could play, I found myself wondering if I'd bitten off more than I could chew; he's a sadist. And there were times over the next months when I had to make difficult adjustments and wondered if it wasn't more than I wanted to deal with. But never seriously so, and each time the rightness of the relationship reasserted itself.

There was luck involved. I'd made my initial decisions about him three years before I actually met him. I wasn't ready when I first saw that he was looking for a slave, and when I was ready, I'd assumed that surely, by then, he would have found one, so I didn't even consider him. It was after a failed attempt with someone else that I stumbled across another of his ads, in a resource I had deliberately tried to ignore.

Sir: How has your commitment changed over the years?

It's a given that relationships change with time because people change and grow as well. If a relationship is to continue the people involved have to adjust to each other's changes and growth, in ways that continue to be supportive of the other while maintaining the right to grow as well. That's what commitment is.

When you go through the rough times without taking potshots at each other...difficulty, illness, depression, money issues... turmoil can strengthen a relationship by making it pliable, thereby helping it weather greater turmoil. When stress occurs on one side and the other offers support, greater trust develops allowing the stress to be weathered. When each finds happiness in the other's growth without letting it stifle their own, satisfaction with life increases. All of these things cause the commitment to change, and when the change is positive the relationship remains strong and gets better.

Has our commitment changed over the years? Certainly it has. Turmoil, stress, support, trust, satisfaction...have all strengthened our relationship because we have approached it together in realistic and positive ways.

Sir: How did you get trained to be a slave?
First I had to find out what exactly was meant by slavery and that wasn't exactly easy to do. The art and stories made it look "hot" but I'd had enough life experience to know that "hot" took a lot of energy to maintain and it isn't a constant state. Then I had to explore it and learn the difference between leather, S&M, bondage, and master/slave relationships. Many, newcomers especially and those who haven't taken the time to really explore what master/slave is really about, think it's all part and parcel of the same thing. They all relate to one another but they are not the same thing, and learning the differences, and how I enjoyed each activity, helped me come to know what I really wanted. S&M can be erotic and sexy and fun, but it's more so when it takes place in the context of the type of dominance and submission that a master/slave relationship provides. Maybe it's the difference between chocolate flavoring and real chocolate.

Once I knew what I liked and why, and how I most enjoyed it, I was then able to begin exploring how being a slave fit me and into the life I wanted. I got my head around the idea and what it meant so I could devote my energy towards it. Though many people provided the means to learn this I guess I was "self-trained". Once I found a master the specific training occurred, learning how he prefers my service to take place. So while I might know a variety of different protocols I learned what ones he wanted me to practice. This is often the hardest lesson a slave has to learn... letting the Master be served the way THEY want to be served.

Sir: Do you ever have to train Jack?
Well, he's trainable, but sometimes it isn't easy. And sometimes he just refuses to learn.

It isn't a slave's place to make their master or mistress into who they want them to be, though many slave wannabes carry the very same illusion that many typical "couples" enter a relationship with: "They'll change to be who I want them to be". And when they don't succeed (as befalls many typical couples as well) they appear surprised, as though the reality is supposed to be different for them. The foolish wannabe will let love-at-first-sight blind them long before a blindfold or hood does.

Control is what defines a master/slave relationship; success is realizing who controls whom and who should control what. But any master or mistress worth their salt will understand that they have to sacrifice some of their fantasies and routines, in their own way and on their own terms. A slave adapts to their Master's lifestyle and a smart slave wannabe has enough foresight to see potential problems before they arise.

I can think of only of two or three instances in ten years where it could be said I "trained" Sir to my will. Who knows? He might just be biding his time. He gets his way, tempered by logic, understanding, acknowledgement, patience and perseverance, and adjustments where needed.

Sir: What does punishment mean to you?
It means separation. It's an emotional or spiritual act rather than a physical act. The physical act of punishment is merely a symbol; it wipes the slate clean and puts the guilt aside. It's a way of removing the separation so the relationship can move forward again. Failure occurs but the act of punishment and a spirit of doing better allows for growth.

Sir uses a brush as the punishment tool, but it isn't the tool itself that creates the real pain. It's the knowledge that he's had to turn to that to make his point. The same tool can be used in play without the same meaning.

One of the more difficult things is to try to explain the concept of punishment to someone not involved in such a relationship. It seems silly. "Adults don't punish each other in such overt ways." so trying to explain it just doesn't work well. Actually, adults do punish, often in cruel and on-going ways that do far more damage to a relationship than it helps. Far better, I think, is the act of punishment and acceptance that takes place in a master/slave relationship.

Sir: Are there any details in your relationship that are especially important?
Communication and honesty are the core values of our relationship. They make everything else possible and allow our energy to be given to the productive side of our relationship.

So is the constant affirmation of our relationship and the place each of us has in it. Sir's notoriety plays an important role, as well. Not in that he is well known but that our relationship tends to be so public and that plays a role in it as well.

Not unique to us is that the level of dominance and submission breeds a closeness, and an ability to seemingly know what the other is thinking. Focusing on another so intimately means there is a constant subconscious feedback that clues you in on each other. It reinforces a sense of oneness. Traditional marriage sees this happening quite often early in the marriage but as other responsibilities get in the way those clues often go unnoticed. Domination/submission helps maintain the focus.

Sir: How do you manage to be active at work, in your clubs, and still be a slave?

Not very well I'm afraid. They all have the ability to take away my focus from Sir from time to time and it's very discouraging for me when I realize that's happened. There are many times when I want to go back to that time when nothing interested me more than getting to suck that cock and figuring ways to put Sir on a pedestal.

Focusing energy creatively on something other than Sir has a tendency to shift my focus away from Sir, whether it's work, volunteering, etc., anything that isn't being done specifically for Sir. It's frustrating but it occurs, and it has made me grow as a person.

Submission often involves turning over control of your creativity, and that can give an aura of being unable to think for yourself. That comes as part of the initial training where you are surrendering everything, all control, and learning to follow your master's lead. Once that surrender is a part of you it can be important (depending upon your master's preferences) to make room for initiative and creativity once again in order to maintain mental health, and, ultimately, the health of the relationship.

But often others who don't understand the relationship go on the assumption that you are incapable of managing yourself and making your own decisions when necessary. Early on I began using the phrase "I'm submissive, not stupid" as a way of indicating that I am still a functioning human being.

Sir: What is sex like for you?

Good, most times; frustrating sometimes; occasionally inconvenient. I think the nature of the relationship makes it consistently more erotic. The dominance/submission dynamic, particularly the surrendering, creates a special energy that drives the sex.

For us sex, occurs practically daily, though that's going to depend on the drive and energy of the individuals involved. In essence, it's going to depend upon the importance they put on sex in the relationship. It doesn't happen all of the time, though that's what many wannabes think they want it to be like, and for many, it's the core of why they think they want to be a slave.

Because the dominance/submission is 24/7/365, there is an underlying sexually that does linger throughout the day. It's reinforced by the rituals and protocols we practice, by his patting me on the ass or walking up to me and embracing and holding me until I stop and give in, or when

I wander over and nuzzle Sir's crotch (I know from experience that it is okay for me to initiate this. He maintains the control by grabbing my head and holding it, by pushing me away either at the beginning or when he's ready for me to stop, or by encouraging me on to more than nuzzling), by my service and obedience (and his expecting service and obedience), and by many other little actions or behaviors that freely occur in this type of "no permission needed" on his part and the letting go and accepting on my part of the relationship.

The main thing is that we don't let sex embarrass us. We aren't shy about it, we don't apologize for it, and we see it as a part of our everyday routine.

Sir: Do you ever mind that Jack has other slaves and tricks?

No. I feel secure in my relationship with Sir and others being around doesn't threaten me. How I serve Sir is unique and special and he readily acknowledges it. All anyone else can do is enhance what I already give him.

Sir: So, is being a slave really good for you?

Without question. Before I became Sir's slave there was always this sense that I was pretending in life, which led to a lack of confidence and an uncertainty. I knew no one would understand who I wanted to be so I had to keep it a secret and this created an enormous sense of loneliness that lingered in other parts of my life. Loneliness breeds stress, and poor health, and dissatisfaction. I've found a great strength in being able to live out who I really am. Life really becomes worth living and suddenly it's worth living well.

Sir: Don't you wish you had a lover?

No, I don't. My relationship with Sir is important to me in ways that a lover relationship could never be. I think it would be unfair, as well, to give a lover or second Master less than my full energy and effort. There are times when I can barely do that for Sir. Particularly in a 24/7/365 master/slave relationship, divided loyalties will always end up with one or the other getting less than they should have.

Appendix E:

Resources

BOOKS

This reading list only represents titles specific to the subject of master/ slave relationships, kinky sex as it relates to M/s relationships, or personal growth topics intended to add to your skills as a slave. For a more complete listings of books dealing with our lifestyle please visit resources such as www.KinkyBooks.com.

Abernathy, Christina, Miss Abernathy's Concise Slave Training Manual, Greenery Press, 1996. [0963976397]

Abernathy, Christina, Training with Miss Abernathy: A Workbook for Erotic Slaves and Their Owners, Greenery Press, 1998. [1890159077]

Allen, Robert (Daddy Bob), The Wings of Icarus, Robert A. Allen Publishing, 1996. [096551000X]

Anapol, Dr. Deborah M, Polyamory, The New Love without Limit, Intinet Resource Center, 1997. [1880789086]

Antoniou, Laura, The Marketplace Series, Books 1-5, Mystic Rose Press, 2000 - 2003. Various ISBN numbers.

Baldwin, Guy, SlaveCraft: Roadmaps for Erotic Servitude, Principles, Skills and Tools, Daedalus Publishing, 2002. [1881943143]

Guy Baldwin, Joseph W. Bean, Joseph Bean (Editor), Ties That Bind: The SM/Leather/Fetish Erotic Style: Issues, Commentaries and Advice, Daedalus Publishing, 1993. [1881943097]

Easton, Dossie, and Catherine A. Liszt, The Ethical Slut, a Guide to Infinite Sexual Possibilities, Greenery Press, 1997. [1890159018]

Hendrix, Harville, Getting the Love You Want, The Institute for Imago Relationship Therapy, 1997 [1880789086]

Johnson, V. M, To Love, To Obey, To Serve: Diary of an Old Guard Slave, Mystic Rose Books, 1999. [0964596024]

Kiersey, David and Marilyn Bates, Please Understand Me, Character and Temperament Types, Prometheus Nemesis, 1978. [0960695400] McKay, Matthew, Messages: The Communication Skills Book, New Harbinger Publishing, 1983. [0934986053]

Preston, John, Mr. Benson. Cleis Press, 2004. [1573441945]

Puppy Sharon and Steven Toushin, Puppy Papers: A Woman's Journey Life and Journey into BDSM, Wells Street Pub., 2004. [1884760031]

Rinella, Jack, Partners in Power, Living In Kinky Relationships, Greenery Press, 2003. [1890159506]

Rinella, Jack, The Compleat Slave, Creating and Maintaining an Erotic Dominant/submissive Relationship, Daedalus Publishing, 2002. [1881943143]

Rinella, Jack, The Master's Manual, A Handbook of Erotic Dominance, Daedalus Publishing, 1994. [1881943038]

Stein, David, Carried Away: An S/M Romance, Daedalus Publishing, 2002. [1881943178]

ORGANIZATIONS:
A short listing of SM-related organizations specific to our lifestyle.

The Leather Archives and Museum at 6418 North Greenview, Chicago, 60626, (773) 761-9200 http://www.leatherarchives.org "Located in Chicago and serving the world," this museum provides educational services to those interested in our community's history. Writings, leather, SM, Fetish, Motorcycle memorabilia from around the world.

MAsT (Masters And slaves Together) "is an organization for adults who live the dominant/submissive lifestyle." MAsT chapters are located in major metropolitan areas and in many smaller cities. Chapters vary in orientation, sexual preference, style of organization, and activities. More information can be found at their website: http://www.mast. net.

NCFS (National Coalition for Sexual Freedom) at http://www. ncsfreedom.org is our national resource for legal information about SM. They monitor mainstream news coverage and legal affairs as they may relate to our community and offer assistance to groups and individuals in need of legal counsel and advice.

National Domestic Violence Hotline toll-free at 800-799-SAFE (800-799-7233). http://www.ndvh.org. "The Hotline provides crisis intervention, information about domestic violence and referrals to local, state, and national resources to which both the abused and abusers can turn. For victims of domestic violence and those calling on their behalf."

INTERNET RESOURCES:
Of the innumerable websites and Internet resources available to our lifestyle, I've included a short listing of my personal favorites:

Kink Aware Professionals (http://www.bannon.com/kap) is a resource for finding medical, legal, financial, and technical professionals who are informed about the diversity of consensual, adult sexuality.

LeatherPage (http//:www.leatherpage.com) carries weekly columns on our lifestyle including Mr. Marcus, Lolita, Cain Berlinger, and others.

KinkyBooks (http://www.kinkybooks.com) An online bookstore offering more than 700 titles specially selected for our community.

LeatherViews (http://www.leatherviews.com) is my own website and features a full collection of my writing, links, and biographical data.

EVENTS:
Our community has numerous events across the company and at each of them you will find members of and workshops specific to our lifestyle. Below are events specific to master/slave relationship:

International Master and Slave Contest at South Plains LeatherFest happens each year in late February in Dallas. The contest, along with a workshop emphasis focused on master/slave relationships is the largest gathering of those involved in our lifestyle. More information at their website http://www.southplainsleatherfest.com

Great Lakes Master and slave Contest at Great Lakes Leather Alliance Weekend takes place in late summer each year in Indianapolis, IN. Their website is located at http://www.greatlakesleather.org

Master/slave Conference, the regional Northeast Master/slave Contest, takes place in late summer each year in Washington, D.C. Visit their website at http://www.masterslaveconference.org for more information.

Southwest Master/slave Contest at Southwest Leather Conference takes place each year in Phoenix, AZ. Visit their web site: http://www.southwestleather.org for additional information.

Together in Leather and Southeast Master/slave Contest take place in Charlotte, NC in October of each year. Their website provides further information on the events: http://www.togetherinleather.org

Weekend Training Events:
As of this writing I have information on the following training events that focus on master/slave relationships. All are safe, sane, consensual environments with experienced, knowledgeable facilitators:

APEX Academy Butchmanns Tradition in Phoenix is hosted four times a year and brings together some of the premier leather leaders in the country to celebrate and develop the collective heart and spirit we all share as Leatherfolk. (http://www.arizonapowerexchange.org/academy)

Jack Rinella's Master & slave Training Institute is an intensive small group weekend seminar for would-be masters and slaves that discusses and explores the topics in this book in workshop, discussion and small group sessions. (http://www.LeatherViews.com),

Master Taino's Training Academy in Washington, DC. has separate slave training and Master training sessions aimed at those who have little or no experience in BDSM and master/slave relationships and those struggling to define their true feelings and identity as submissive men or dominants. (http://www.mastertaino.com/slave_training.htm)

Master's Retreat "The Retreat is open to anyone who identifies as Daddy, Master, or Mistress, regardless of sexual orientation or gender, and who desires to be served by a boy, boi, submissive, or slave. Experience with or possession of a submissive is not a requirement for attending. (http://www.LeatherNetwork.com)

Boy's Training Camp (bTC) brings together those who identify as submissive, regardless of sexual orientation or gender, who desire to serve. Participants engage in training, an exchange of knowledge and information, and peer support. Experience or being in service to a dominant is not required (http://www.LeatherNetwork.com)

Servant's Retreat "SR is about using tools to be a whole person and bringing the power of everything you are into service. At Retreat, we will explore in depth who we are as servants/bottoms/slaves/boys/ girls/and people." (http://www.bdsmclasses.com)

About the Author

Jack Rinella is the author of *The Master's Manual, The Compleat slave, The Toy Bag Guide to Clips and Clamps,* and *Partners In Power.* He is a freelance writer and college instructor.

Jack has been an active participant in BDSM for more than 20 years, ten years of which he has been the master of his 24/7 slave Patrick and five years of which he lived as a slave in service to Master Lynn.

He started his career as a writer of kinky columns in 1992 when he began writing his weekly column LeatherViews, which still appears in Gay Chicago Magazine. His columns have also appeared in Philadelphia, San Francisco, via email and on the World Wide Web.

He is an active member of the Chicago Hellfire Club, a founding member of Masters And slaves Together - Chicago, and on the board of directors of the Leather Leadership Conference, Inc.

Born in upstate New York of Italian-American parents, he's been a high school and college teacher, a drug rehabilitation counselor, a cook, a computer salesman, a Catholic seminarian, a Pentecostal minister, an advertising copy writer, a graphic designer, and has done stints at printing, publishing, telemarketing, head-hunting, and computer consulting. He lives on the North side of Chicago where he passes the time writing, cruising, and falling in love whenever he can. You can contact Jack at mrjackr@Leathermail.com.

Also by Jack Rinella
Available from KinkyBooks.com
www.KinkyBooks.com 800-932-7111
1363 N. Wells Street Chicago, IL 60610
Celebrating Healthy Sexuality!

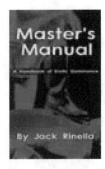 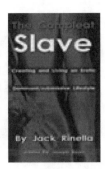 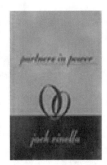 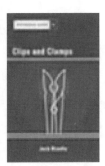

The Master's Manual: A Handbook of Erotic Dominance
$15.95 1994 ISBN:1881943038, Daedalus Publishing, 199 Pages.
Jack Rinella's best-selling Handbook of Erotic Dominance. Does domination of another turn you on? Examines various aspects of erotic dominance, including SM, safety, sex. Erotic power, techniques, and much more.

The Compleat Slave: Creating and Living an Erotic Dominant/submissive Relationship $15.95 2001 ISBN:1881943135, Daedalus Publishing, 176 Pages. Jack Rinella continues his in-depth exploration and discussion of Dominant/submissive relationships. Features Rinella's guidelines, tips, and personal experiences in creating safe and sane Master/slave relationships.

Partners In Power: Living In kinky Relationships $16.95 2003 ISBN:1890159530, Greenery Press, 203 Pages. Erotic sex is all about deeper relationships and this is the first relationship book written specifically for the kink community. It covers all kinds of relationships and the issues that come up with making them work. Anyone seeking a deeper understanding of the complexity of BDSM relationships can learn a great deal from "Partners in Power."

The Toybag Guide to Clips and Clamps $9.95 2004 ISBN:1890159557, Greenery Press, 127 Pages. A quick reference guide to everything pinchy, from simple wooden clothespins to hand-tooled precision devices of gleaming chrome. Clamps offer a versatile spectrum of sensation to the knowledgeable player, and this book is the clamp-user's best friend. Advice, suggestions, and basic safety tips.

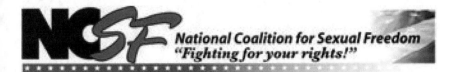
The National Coalition for Sexual Freedom

The National Coalition for Sexual Freedom (NCSF) is a national organization committed to altering the political, legal, and social environment in the United States in order to guarantee equal rights for consenting adults who practice forms of alternative sexual expression. NCSF is primarily focused on the rights of consenting adults in the SM-Leather-fetish, swing and polyamory communities, who often face discrimination because of their sexual expression.

Did you know...Your private sexual expression can be used against you:

- **People like you lose child custody because of their interest in the Lifestyle.**

- **People like you lose their jobs because swinging and polyamory violate morality clauses.**

- **People like you lose your clubs because religious extremists and conservative politicians zone sexual activities out of your city.**

Are you going to let them tell you how to live your life?

Contact NCSF if you have a problem or want to help us with our work:

National Coalition for Sexual Freedom
822 Guilford Avenue, Box 127
Baltimore, MD 21202-3707
E-mail: ncsfreedom@ncsfreedom.org
phone: 410-539-4824
fax: 410-385-2827

301